79.95

Health Informatics
(formerly Computers in Health Care)

Kathryn J. Hannah   Marion J. Ball
Series Editors

For other titles published in this series, go to
www.springer.com/series/1114

Laura Einbinder · Nancy M. Lorenzi
Joan S. Ash · Cynthia S. Gadd
Jonathan Einbinder
Editors

Transforming Health Care Through Information: Case Studies

Third Edition

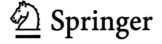 Springer

Editors

Laura Einbinder
Partners Health Care
Center for Clinical Informatics
    Research and Development
Research Applications Group
Boston, MA,
USA

Nancy M. Lorenzi
Vanderbilt University Medical Center
Department of Biomedical Informatics
Eskind Biomedical Library 4th floor
2209 Garland Avenue
Nashville, TN 37232-8340
USA

Joan S. Ash
Oregon Health Science University
Department of Medical Informatics
    & Clinical Epidemiology
3181 SW Sam Jackson Park Road
Mailcode: BICC
Portland, OR 97239–3098

Cynthia S. Gadd
Vanderbilt University Medical Center
Department of Biomedical Informatics
Eskind Biomedical Library 4th floor
2209 Garland Avenue
Nashville, TN 37232–8340
USA

Jonathan Einbinder
Partners Health Care
Center for Clinical Informatics
    Research and Development
Research Applications Group
Boston, MA
USA

ISBN 978-1-4419-0268-9   e-ISBN 978-1-4419-0269-6
DOI 10.1007/978-1-4419-0269-6
Springer New York Dordrecht Heidelberg London

Library of Congress Control Number: 2009931684

Printed on acid-free paper

Springer is part of Springer Science+Business Media (www.springer.com)

*My dedication is to Robert T. Riley,
the managing editor of the first edition
of Transforming Health Care through
Information: Case Studies. In that role he
edited all the cases and ensured that they
were more readable and had a sense
of balance and humor. Bob was nationally and
internationally acclaimed for his presentations,
his management developmental seminars,
and his consulting skills. He authored
several books and numerous articles on
management and on managing technological
change. Bob was known for his humor, his
constant quest for new knowledge, his ability
to understand and solve problems, his ability to
make friends, and his ability to teach
others. By publishing yet another edition in
this series, we continue to remember and
honor his memory.*

Foreword

By any measure, our field of clinical informatics is poised for rapid growth and expansion. A confluence of forces and trends, including pressure to contain health care costs and simultaneously expand access and coverage, a desire to reduce medical error and health care disparities, the need to better understand and optimize our clinical interventions and delivery systems, the need to translate new knowledge into practice quickly and effectively, and the need to demonstrate the value of our services, all call for the application of the methods and techniques of our field – some of which are well honed with experience, and some of which are still in the process of being discovered. Clinical informatics is not the only solution to what ails health care, but it is a critical component of the solution.

Our methods and techniques are similar in many ways to the knowledge base of any interdisciplinary field: some are informed by experience, the trials and tribulations of figuring out what works through real world implementation, some are informed by controlled experimentation in randomized controlled trials and related studies, some are informed by critical observation and analysis, and some are developed through laboratory evaluation rather than field trials. As we develop both the basic science, as well as the applied science, of our field, there is a critical role for learning from others by way of case reports and stories. These reports of work in progress contribute in significant ways to the growing understanding of what works, and what does not, in practice. They play a key role in helping to develop and evolve a framework of understanding, on which we may hang a variety of evidence to substantiate, or to reform our principles and theory, and with which we may identify the key questions that are yet to be assessed.

The following text is a collection of case reports and stories, some more formal than others, but all contributing to this evolving framework of understanding, and all of which will help any practitioner in the field of clinical informatics increase his or her understanding, and become better able to pursue their own trials and tribulations with any clinical informatics project, and contribute their own experiences to the framework. The text is organized around four major areas or domains of clinical informatics – Managing Change, Patient Safety, Organizational Impact and Evaluation, and Integration – and focuses on the people and organizational process of applied informatics, as well as evaluation, across a wide range of topics. The authors are all deeply involved in their projects and they bring an intimate understanding of the problems at hand. The editors are all expert leaders in the field, who have brought these authors together and created this rich collection. These stories will inform, entertain, surprise, and console the reader – we have much to offer in our field, but we may be humbled by the scope of the challenge, and we will surely benefit from sharing our stories and insights.

Read and enjoy this book – and learn from it more about what works, and what may not work in practice, and apply it to your own efforts. Your own understanding will be much improved, and you will be more likely to succeed. And, in any case, you will add your own experience to the framework of understanding. Be sure to write your story, too.

Partners Healthcare System   Blackford Middleton, MD, MPH, MSc
Wellesley, MA

Series Preface

This series is directed to Health care professionals who are leading the transformation of health care by using information and knowledge. Historically the series was launched in 1988 as Computers in Health Care, to offer a broad range of titles: some addressed to specific professions such as nursing, medicine, and health administration; others to special areas of practice such as trauma and radiology; still other books in the series focused on interdisciplinary issues, such as the computer based patient record, electronic health records, and networked Health care systems. Renamed Health Informatics in 1998 to reflect the rapid evolution in the discipline known as health Informatics, the series continued to add titles that contribute to the evolution of the field. In the series, eminent experts, serving as editors or authors, offer their accounts of innovations in health Informatics. Increasingly, these accounts go beyond hardware and software to address the role of information in influencing the transformation of Health care delivery systems around the world. The series also increasingly focused on the users of the information and systems: the organizational, behavioral, and societal changes that accompany the diffusion of information technology in health services environments.

Developments in health care delivery are constant; most recently developments in proteomics and genomics are increasingly becoming relevant to clinical decision making and emerging standards of care. The data resources emerging from molecular biology are beyond the capacity of the human brain to integrate and beyond the scope of paper based decision trees. Thus, bioinformatics has emerged as a new field in health informatics to support emerging and ongoing developments in molecular biology. Translational informatics supports acceleration, from bench to bedside, i.e. the appropriate use of molecular biology research findings and bioinformatics in clinical care of patients.

At the same time, further continual evolution of the field of Health informatics is reflected in the introduction of concepts at the macro or health systems delivery level with major national initiatives related to electronic health records (EHR), data standards and public health informatics such as the Health care Information Technology Standards Panel (HITSP) in the United States, Canada Health Infoway, NHS Connecting for Health in the UK.

We have consciously retained the series title Health Informatics as the single umbrella term that encompasses both the microscopic elements of bioinformatics and the macroscopic aspects of large national health information systems. Ongoing changes to both the micro and macro perspectives on health informatics will continue to shape health services in the twenty-first century. By making full and creative use of the technology to tame data and to transform information, health Informatics will foster the development and use of new knowledge in health care. As coeditors, we pledge to support our professional colleagues and the series readers as they share advances in the emerging and exciting field of Health Informatics.

Kathryn J. Hannah
Marion J. Ball

Acknowledgments

To students in my class who investigated the people and organizational issues side of informatics.

Nancy M. Lorenzi

Contents

Section I   Managing Change
Nancy M. Lorenzi

1   **Back Breaking Work: Implementing
    a Spine Registry in an Orthopedic Clinic** 7
    Brian C. Drolet

2   **A RHIO Struggling to Form: Will it Get Off the Ground?** 15
    Paul Zlotnik, Denny Lee, Mike Minear, and Prashila Dullabh

3   **A Rough Ride at the Theodore Roosevelt Cancer Center** 29
    Karen Albert, Nitika Gupta, Teresa Mason, and Purvi Mehta

4   **Implementation of an Electronic Prescription Writer
    in Ambulatory Care** 47
    Minhui Xie and Kevin B. Johnson

5   **Online Health Care: A Classic Clash of Technology,
    People and Processes** 57
    John Butler, Dan Dalan, Brian McCourt, John Norris,
    and Randall Stewart

Section II   Patient Safety
Joan S. Ash

6   **A Dungeon of Dangerous Practices** 73
    Andrew Amata, Allen Flynn, Michelle Morgan,
    Teresa Smith, and Mary Tengdin

7   **Different Sides of the Story** 83
    Allison B. McCoy

8   **Barcode Medication Administration Implementation
    in the FIAT Health System** 85
    Linda Chan, William Greeley, Don Klingen,
    Brian Machado, Michael Padula, John Sum, and Angela Vacca

9   **H.I.T. or Miss** 97
    James McCormack, Bimal R. Desai, Jennifer Garvin,
    Randal Hamric, Kirk Lalwani, Andi Lushaj, Alexey Panchenko,
    Deborah Quitmeyer, and JoAnna M. Vanderhoef

Section III   Organizational Impact and Evaluation
Cynthia S. Gadd

10 **The Implementation of Secure Messaging** 107
    Zhou Yan

11 **Who Moved My Clinic? Donnelly University
    Pediatric Rehabilitation: The Wheelchair Clinic** 115
    Fredrick Hilliard

12 **OncoOrders: The Early Years** 127
    Chris Raggio and Judith W. Dexheimer

13 **Implementing a Computerized Triage System
    in the Emergency Department** 135
    Scott R. Levin, Daniel J. France, and Dominik Aronsky

14 **Medication Barcode Scanning: Code "Moo": Dead COW** 155
    Laurie L. Novak and Kathy S. Moss

Section IV   Integration
Jonathan S. Einbinder

15 **Project NEED: New Efficiency
    in an Emergency Department** 167
    Barry Little, Denise Johnson, Jennifer Tingle,
    Mary Stanfill, and Michael Roy

16 **Digital Radiology Divide at McKinly** 179
    Neal Goldstein, David Ross, Ken Christensen,
    Jayashree Kalpathy-Cramer, Aseem Kumar,
    and Marilyn Schroeder

Index 191

Contributors

Karen Albert
Department of Medical Informatics & Clinical Epidemiology, Oregon Health
Science University, Portland, OR 97239-3098, USA

Andrew Amata
Department of Medical Informatics & Clinical Epidemiology, Oregon Health
Science University, Portland, OR 97239-3098, USA

Dominik Aronsky
Eskind Biomedical Library, Departments of Biomedical Informatics and
Emergency Medicine, Vanderbilt University Medical Center, Nashville,
TN 37232-8340, USA

Joan S. Ash
Department of Medical Informatics & Clinical Epidemiology, Oregon Health
Science University, Portland, OR 97239-3098, USA

John Butler
Department of Medical Informatics & Clinical Epidemiology, Oregon Health
Science University, Portland, OR 97239-3098, USA

Linda Chan
Department of Medical Informatics & Clinical Epidemiology, Oregon Health
Science University, Portland, OR 97239-3098, USA

Ken Christensen
Department of Medical Informatics & Clinical Epidemiology, Oregon Health
Science University, Portland, OR 97239-3098, USA

Dan Dalan
Department of Medical Informatics & Clinical Epidemiology, Oregon Health
Science University, Portland, OR 97239-3098, USA

Bimal R. Desai
Department of Medical Informatics & Clinical Epidemiology, Oregon Health
Science University, Portland, OR 97239-3098, USA

Judith W. Dexheimer
Eskind Biomedical Library, Department of Biomedical Informatics, Vanderbilt
University Medical Center, Nashville, TN 37232-8340, USA

Brian C. Drolet
Eskind Biomedical Library, Department of Biomedical Informatics, Vanderbilt
University Medical Center, Nashville, TN 37232-8340, USA

Prashila Dullabh
Department of Medical Informatics & Clinical Epidemiology, Oregon Health
Science University, Portland, OR 97239-3098, USA

Jonathan S. Einbinder
Research Applications Group, Center for Clinical Informatics Research and
Development, Partners Health Care, Boston, MA, USA

Laura Einbinder
Research Applications Group, Center for Clinical Informatics Research and
Development, Partners Health Care, Boston, MA, USA

Allen Flynn
Department of Medical Informatics & Clinical Epidemiology, Oregon Health
Science University, Portland, OR 97239-3098, USA

Daniel J. France
Eskind Biomedical Library, Departments of Biomedical Engineering and
Anesthesia, Vanderbilt University Medical Center, Nashville, TN 37232-8340,
USA

Cynthia S. Gadd
Eskind Biomedical Library, Department of Biomedical Informatics, Vanderbilt
University Medical Center, Nashville, TN 37232-8340, USA

Jennifer Garvin
Department of Medical Informatics & Clinical Epidemiology, Oregon Health
Science University, Portland, OR 97239-3098, USA

Neal Goldstein
Department of Medical Informatics & Clinical Epidemiology, Oregon Health
Science University, Portland, OR 97239-3098, USA

William Greeley
Department of Medical Informatics & Clinical Epidemiology, Oregon Health
Science University, Portland, OR 97239-3098, USA

Nitika Gupta
Department of Medical Informatics & Clinical Epidemiology, Oregon Health
Science University, Portland, OR 97239-3098, USA

Randal Hamric
Department of Medical Informatics & Clinical Epidemiology, Oregon Health
Science University, Portland, OR 97239-3098, USA

Fredrick Hilliard
Eskind Biomedical Library, Department of Biomedical Informatics, Vanderbilt
University Medical Center, Nashville, TN 37232-8340, USA

Denise Johnson
Department of Medical Informatics & Clinical Epidemiology, Oregon Health
Science University, Portland, OR 97239-3098, USA

Kevin B. Johnson
Eskind Biomedical Library, Department of Biomedical Informatics, Vanderbilt
University Medical Center, Nashville, TN 37232-8340, USA

Jayashree Kalpathy-Cramer
Department of Medical Informatics & Clinical Epidemiology, Oregon Health
Science University, Portland, OR 97239-3098, USA

Don Klingen
Department of Medical Informatics & Clinical Epidemiology, Oregon Health
Science University, Portland, OR 97239-3098, USA

Aseem Kumar
Department of Medical Informatics & Clinical Epidemiology, Oregon Health
Science University, Portland, OR 97239-3098, USA

Kirk Lalwani
Department of Medical Informatics & Clinical Epidemiology, Oregon Health
Science University, Portland, OR 97239-3098, USA

Denny Lee
Department of Medical Informatics & Clinical Epidemiology, Oregon Health
Science University, Portland, OR 97239-3098, USA

Scott R. Levin
Department of Emergency Medicine, Johns Hopkins University, Baltimore, MD,
21287 USA

Barry Little
Department of Medical Informatics & Clinical Epidemiology, Oregon Health
Science University, Portland, OR 97239-3098, USA

Nancy M. Lorenzi
Eskind Biomedical Library, Department of Biomedical Informatics, Vanderbilt
University Medical Center, Nashville, TN 37232-8340, USA

Andi Lushaj
Department of Medical Informatics & Clinical Epidemiology, Oregon Health
Science University, Portland, OR 97239-3098, USA

Brian Machado
Department of Medical Informatics & Clinical Epidemiology, Oregon Health
Science University, Portland, OR 97239-3098, USA

Teresa Mason
Department of Medical Informatics & Clinical Epidemiology, Oregon Health
Science University, Portland, OR 97239-3098, USA

James McCormack
Department of Medical Informatics & Clinical Epidemiology, Oregon Health
Science University, Portland, OR 97239-3098, USA

Brian McCourt
Department of Medical Informatics & Clinical Epidemiology, Oregon Health
Science University, Portland, OR 97239-3098, USA

Allison B. McCoy
Eskind Biomedical Library, Department of Biomedical Informatics, Vanderbilt
University Medical Center, Nashville, TN 37232-8340, USA

Purvi Mehta
Department of Medical Informatics & Clinical Epidemiology, Oregon Health
Science University, Portland, OR 97239-3098, USA

Mike Minear
Department of Medical Informatics & Clinical Epidemiology, Oregon Health
Science University, Portland, OR 97239-3098, USA

Michelle Morgan
Department of Medical Informatics & Clinical Epidemiology, Oregon Health
Science University, Portland, OR 97239-3098, USA

Kathy S. Moss
Eskind Biomedical Library, Department of Biomedical Informatics, Vanderbilt
University Medical Center, Nashville, TN 37232-8340, USA

John Norris
Department of Medical Informatics & Clinical Epidemiology, Oregon Health
Science University, Portland, OR 97239-3098, USA

Laurie L. Novak
Eskind Biomedical Library, Department of Biomedical Informatics, Vanderbilt
University Medical Center, Nashville, TN 37232-8340, USA

Michael Padula
Department of Medical Informatics & Clinical Epidemiology, Oregon Health
Science University, Portland, OR 97239-3098, USA

Alexey Panchenko
Department of Medical Informatics & Clinical Epidemiology, Oregon Health
Science University, Portland, OR 97239-3098, USA

Deborah Quitmeyer
Department of Medical Informatics & Clinical Epidemiology, Oregon Health
Science University, Portland, OR 97239-3098, USA

Chris Raggio
Eskind Biomedical Library, Department of Biomedical Informatics, Vanderbilt
University Medical Center, Nashville, TN 37232-8340, USA

David Ross
Department of Medical Informatics & Clinical Epidemiology, Oregon Health
Science University, Portland, OR 97239-3098, USA

Michael Roy
Department of Medical Informatics & Clinical Epidemiology, Oregon Health
Science University, Portland, OR 97239-3098, USA

Marilyn Schroeder
Department of Medical Informatics & Clinical Epidemiology, Oregon Health
Science University, Portland, OR 97239-3098, USA

Teresa Smith
Department of Medical Informatics & Clinical Epidemiology, Oregon Health
Science University, Portland, OR 97239-3098, USA

Mary Stanfill
Department of Medical Informatics & Clinical Epidemiology, Oregon Health
Science University, Portland, OR 97239-3098, USA

Randall Stewart
Department of Medical Informatics & Clinical Epidemiology, Oregon Health
Science University, Portland, OR 97239-3098, USA

John Sum
Department of Medical Informatics & Clinical Epidemiology, Oregon Health
Science University, Portland, OR 97239-3098, USA

Mary Tengdin
Department of Medical Informatics & Clinical Epidemiology, Oregon Health
Science University, Portland, OR 97239-3098, USA

Jennifer Tingle
Department of Medical Informatics & Clinical Epidemiology, Oregon Health
Science University, Portland, OR 97239-3098, USA

Angela Vacca
Department of Medical Informatics & Clinical Epidemiology, Oregon Health
Science University, Portland, OR 97239-3098, USA

JoAnna M. Vanderhoef
Department of Medical Informatics & Clinical Epidemiology, Oregon Health
Science University, Portland, OR 97239-3098, USA

Minhui Xie
Eskind Biomedical Library, Department of Biomedical Informatics, Vanderbilt
University Medical Center, Nashville, TN 37232-8340, USA

Zhou Yan
Eskind Biomedical Library, Department of Biomedical Informatics, Vanderbilt
University Medical Center, Nashville, TN 37232-8340, USA

P.J. Zlotnik
Department of Medical Informatics & Clinical Epidemiology, Oregon Health
Science University, Portland, OR 97239-3098, USA

Section I
Managing Change

Managing Change 3
   Nancy M. Lorenzi

Chapter 1
Back Breaking Work: Implementing a Spine Registry
   in an Orthopedics Clinic 7
   Brian C. Drolet

Chapter 2
A RHIO Struggling to Form: Will it Get Off the Ground 15
   Paul Zlotnik, Denny Lee, Mike Minear, and Prashila Dullabh

Chapter 3
A Rough Ride at the Theodore Roosevelt Cancer Center 29
   Karen Albert, Nitika Gupta, Teresa Mason, and Purvi Mehta

Chapter 4
Implementation of an Electronic Prescription Writer in Ambulatory Care 47
   Minhui Xie and Kevin B. Johnson

Chapter 5
Online Health Care: A Classic Clash of Technology, People and Processes 57
   John Butler, Dan Dalan, Brian McCourt, John Norris, and Randall Stewart

Managing Change

Nancy M. Lorenzi

Major issues regarding the implementation of informatics-based systems have been known and discussed for a number of years. The concept of effectively managing change or gaining adoption is a cornerstone of the discussions.

Change management is the process by which an organization gets to its future state – the vision. Traditional planning processes delineate the steps on the journey. The role of change management is to facilitate that journey. Therefore, creating change starts with creating a vision for change, and then empowering individuals to act as change agents to attain that vision. The empowered change management agents need plans that are (1) total systems approach, (2) realistic, and (3) future oriented. Change management encompasses the effective strategies and programs to enable the champions to achieve the new vision.

There are a number of common principles that underpin all of the change management strategies. We named these principles "The Magnificent Seven" in the first case book in this series.[1] The principles are:

1. Respect for people: Treating people with respect through honesty and trust is the cornerstone, and with respect for people as the leading force, then all the other principles follow, and enrich this basic respect.
2. Involvement: Involving people is another core principle. If you want people to change, they must not be merely informed about the changes, but they must be involved.
3. Empowerment: Once involved, people must be empowered and energized, and they must move beyond involvement to commitment and adoption.
4. Teamwork: People working together to make changes is essential for success.
5. Customer first: The customer must come first. This principle places the customer/user in central position, and requires those on the inside of the organization to shift their perspective, and view the organization from the external or customer's point of view.
6. Openness to change: Creating a culture that is open to change, as opposed to being a closed and highly structured bureaucratic system is critical for success.
7. Vision oriented: There is a need for an organizational vision that people easily understand, and can explain to others.

Change management is a strategy that consists of a set of processes that can help ensure that something significant, e.g., a concept or an informatics-based system is

3

implemented in an orderly controlled and systematic fashion. The goal is to prepare stakeholders for the transformation, ensure that they are knowledgeable to face change in a dynamic work environment, and ultimately ready to embrace the change.

The aim of effective change management strategies is not to eliminate all resistance, but to understand and manage the process. This includes both acceptance and resistance. Practical experience has shown that change is an on-going process of anticipated, emergent and opportunity-based events that have a fluid and unpredictable nature.

These following strategies have proven effective for us in many situations.[2]

Collecting benchmark data – One step in preparing to implement a new system is to gather accurate performance data for the existing system(s).

Analyzing the benefits – early in the overall process, an accurate cost benefit analysis must be performed from the viewpoint of the physician users – and other major user groups as well. A very valid question for any user is "What's in it for me?"

General organizational climate – if the general organizational climate is relatively negative, attack that problem directly through the use of sound organizational development techniques. Installing an informatics system – no matter how good it may be – will not solve this problem. In fact, the system may be doomed by the negative general climate.

Assess the workflow – the current workflow will need to be assessed, and if needed a redesign team can be established. This team could be an internal multi-disciplinary team with people from the various parts of the organization, for example, clinic operations, the quality office, and the informatics department, etc. This team could analyze the operations, and recommend process improvements.

Champions – an informatics system needs champions. The optimal approach is to identify several *medically-respected* physicians to fulfill this champion role. These people should be integrated into the planning process from the beginning with their advice sought on virtually all aspects of the development and implementation process.

General ownership – developing respected champions is only the first step in building general ownership in the system. The primary twin tools for general ownership are involvement and communication. The single best tool in building ownership is participation in the overall process – planning, design, selection, implementation, etc. – by those that the new system will affect.

Building ownership – the danger is that the participation process often attracts the "amateur techies" in the organization, either by self-selection or by appointment. However, these people may not be high-clout people in the organization. It is critical to have some participation from key power people. In health care organizations, this often translates as people who are highly respected *clinically*.

Rapid implementation – as indicated above, a potential downside of involving people early to build ownership is the waiting period between the early involvement and the actual implementation. Within reason, it is a good strategy to concentrate resources on a limited number of projects to minimize the waiting period for system implementation. This will lessen the efforts needed to rebuild the ownership developed in earlier stages.

Realistic expectations – no matter how good the new informatics system is, it will not improve the quality of the coffee. If the physicians are oversold on what the new system will do, the system is doomed to be regarded as at least a partial failure. This includes setting realistic expectations for the impacts on *initial productivity* during the early implementation stages. It is almost inevitable that productivity will initially decline, no matter how good the system and the preparations for its implementation.

Timely training – getting physicians to participate in informatics training in a traditional classroom sense is notoriously difficult. Any training must be brief, high-quality, closely timed to the point of need, and specifically directed to the physicians' needs. Good training does more than merely build skills. Ideally, education starts the selling process, participation adds enthusiasm, and training is the final opportunity to "close the sale."

Extensive support – with modern software tools, there is no excuse for developing systems without extensive contextual on-line user support written in language that the users can understand. Supplementary written support should also be provided in a format most comfortable for the users. When the system is first installed, ample on-site help should be available, to be subsequently replaced with good phone support as the initial demands dwindle. Time-conscious physicians demand prompt, high-quality support, or they rapidly become discontented with the system.

System stability – physicians are busy people. Even if they are willing to invest the time to learn the system, they almost certainly will not be willing to spend the time to relearn the release of the month. Well-crafted software is relatively stable, at least in its user interface, and effective prototyping should sharply limit the number of changes necessary in the interface. There will be bugs, but correcting them should not require constantly modifying the user interface.

Protecting professional egos – although it is costly, skilled one-on-one or very small-group training may be an effective strategy for those physicians, and other professionals most likely to be affected by computer-phobia.

Professionals have an understandable need for respect. Therefore, the dialogues present in informatics systems should be carefully reviewed for usefulness, clarity, and respectful tone. For example, alerts should be programmed as respectful questions rather than as terse declarative statements. Error messages must give useful instructions for correcting the situation.

Feedback processes – any aggressive change management strategy should contain multiple mechanisms for actively soliciting feedback at all stages of the change process. The alternative is to have rumors, half-truths, and even untruths flooding the grapevine. When feedback is solicited and obtained, it must be processed promptly, and return feedback provided. Every issue cannot be resolved to everyone's satisfaction. People must feel that both they and their concerns are regarded as important.

Having fun – smart change managers try to introduce an element of fun into the change management process whenever possible.

Case Introduction

Through the years, we have learned many lessons from change management in large and small settings. There are five cases in this section that continue to illustrate the good, the bad, and the ugly of following or not following the well established change management strategies and practices.

The Drolet case outlines the negotiation skills, and the need for greater buy-in required to gain acceptance of a registry system in an orthopaedic environment. The Zlotnik, Lee, Minear, and Dullabh case illustrates the issues associated with introducing a new system to coordinate and integrate information within a broader region. The Albert, Gupta, Mason, and Mehta case illustrates an implementation of an information system in a more controlled, top-down organizational climate, and the impact of technology on clinical workflow. The Xie and Johnson case focuses on the implementation of one informatics-based product that is also part of an integrated suite of informatics-based products. The Butler, Dalan, McCourt, Norris, and Stewart case focuses on a clash of technology and culture.

All the cases indicate some form of resistance to change, and all case are worth reviewing before your next implementation!

References

1. Lorenzi NM, Riley RT, Ball MJ, Douglas JV. *Transforming Health Care Through Information: Case Studies*. New York: Springer; 1995.
2. Lorenzi NM. Clinical Adoption. In: Lehmann HP, et al., eds. *Aspects of Electronic Health Records*. 2nd ed. New York: Springer; 2006:378-397.

1
Back Breaking Work: Implementing a Spine Registry in an Orthopedic Clinic

Brian C. Drolet

Chris Ryan sighed as he opened an email seeking assistance for yet another technical issue. It was much more than Chris had anticipated when he started the American Spine Registry (ASR) project as a first year medical student 10 months earlier. He had learned a painful lesson through this research experience: implementing a clinical data collection project is anything but simple. Even though Chris had adequate funding and the support of department administration, the project had taken months longer than expected, and each week, it was becoming increasingly more frustrating. At the outset, there were no spoken expectations of technical (computer) expertise or human resource management skills, yet these aspects had consumed more time than any "research" component of the project did. Chris had begun to wonder if he would see this project through to fruition.

Background

The Orthopedic Spine Institute (OSI) is comprised of two spine surgeons practicing within a larger orthopedics department at Lawrence Memorial Medical Center (LMMC), a renowned metropolitan hospital in the southern United States. One of the surgeons, Dr. David Beck, is a recent addition to the faculty, while the other, Dr. Jeffrey Smith, has been in the orthopedic department chair for more than two decades. LMMC is technologically advanced; it uses a state of the art computerized medical record system (Vantage) throughout the hospital. Although the design of Vantage enabled Chris to mine data from the medical documentation, Vantage is a less effective research tool for studying patient data and outcomes.

The spine surgeons are particularly interested in studying the outcomes of their patients so that they can improve their procedures and techniques on the basis of the best available evidence. The surgeons also rely on the data to support their research publications. Prior to this time, the data were either not available or not easily extractable from Vantage. Hence, Chris set out to implement a data collection and storage system outside of Vantage for the explicit purpose of collecting the data required by the surgeons.

The data collection program chosen for the project is called Spine Survey from the ASR. This program administers a modifiable survey for various aspects of patient care including the history of present illness, review of systems, and past medical history. Additionally, Spine Survey utilizes several outcomes measures: the SF-36, Oswestry (Lumbar) Disability Index (ODI), and Neck Disability Index (NDI). [1-3] The survey is

L. Einbinder et al. (eds.), *Transforming Health Care Through Information:* 7
Case Studies, Health Informatics, DOI 10.1007/978-1-4419-0269-6_1,
© Springer Science+Business Media, LLC 2010

logically programmed to prompt questions appropriate for each patient's chief complaint. The patient provides the input to the survey questions using a touch-screen monitor; this information is then directly stored in the local server database. Finally, the surgeon or nurse enters appropriate clinical or operative information for each visit. The plan was to establish an information system separate from Vantage, for the express purpose of research data collection and storage.

Implementation

Chris started his work in October 2005, and he was pleased that Dr. Smith promised him autonomy in his work. Dr. Smith had previously traveled to the east coast to meet with Fred McCoy, the director of the ASR, and had already approved resources – staff and financial – for getting the project underway. Chris started the project by meeting the ASR team by conference call. After conversing several times with Mr. McCoy and viewing PowerPoint presentations sent from the ASR, Chris started feeling moderately comfortable with the Spine Survey data collection software.

In November, a new desktop computer and touch-screen monitor were purchased for use exclusively with Spine Survey. The OSI LAN manager, Edwin Vasquez, insisted on setting up this PC although Chris felt fully capable. The LMMC orthopedics department has dozens of faculty and residents, each with one's own IT needs, and so there were many demands on the LAN manager's time. Unfortunately, Edwin assigned a low priority to the project that was ostensibly under the direction of a first year medical student. Hence, the system was not operational until the middle of December 2005, which of course was right at the start of the several weeks of vacation customarily scheduled for most staff, physicians, and medical students. Consequently, the project was stalled until early January. Chris was eager to get the project moving at the start of the new year. He hoped that the data collection would be up and running in no time.

Finding a suitable location for the computer terminal was the next bump in the road. Since the project involved collecting patient information, privacy was important. The computer was first placed in an empty clinic office, adjacent to the patient waiting room. The office manager, Meredith Jeter, was not at all happy with this setup. She remarked "this office is not free space; it will be used for office expansion." Chris knew immediately that he would have a problem with Ms. Jeter because, in fact, he had been informed that there were no plans to expand the office in the foreseeable future. Despite her protests, it was decided with approval from Dr. Smith that the computer would stay in the empty office as long as the space remained available. Little did he know at the time that winning the support of an office manager would have been very helpful.

About the time that the arrangements were made for the computer terminal placement, Chris learned he would need to secure the computer because of a rash of thefts occurring in the hospital. Because the office space was technically "temporary," a portable, locking computer cabinet was ordered by Edwin. The hospital procurement system caused further delay to the project. It was a memorable day for the staff when the cabinet finally arrived – the cabinet was ugly to say the least. As an unsightly two-tone, metallic-blue and brown, it was oversized at more than six feet height. In the small desktop computer and 17 inch monitor looked comical inside this cavernous locking compartment. To make matters worse, Ms. Jeter was predictably displeased. Setting aside the office manager's concern for esthetics, a real concern was that the monitor shelf was unmovable, which positioned the monitor approximately four feet above the floor. This height made the touch-screen too high for a normal chair. At first, Chris hoped to remedy the situation by obtaining a tall chair so that the patient would be at eye level with the monitor. Pragmatically, the tall chairs are difficult for shorter patients, especially the elderly and those with back or neck injuries, who make up a large portion of OSIs patient population.

Chris continued working with the issues of space, information security, and set up. Meanwhile, the software consultant for the ASR, Jane Maguire, was supposedly working to install Spine Survey through a remote connection. This process ultimately took nearly 5 months. Chris had originally expected to install the software using a CD or DVD like any other program he had used in the past. The remote installation made the process much more complicated than simply "installing" Spine Survey via a CD on the OSI computer.

The first issue was obtaining a secure login into the OSI network for remote access by ASR. Because Jane was connecting from an offsite facility at ASR, getting approval for this access was a lengthy process, which could only be completed by Edwin, who again assigned a low priority to the project. As a result, approval took nearly 2 months. Despite frequent communication with Mr. Vasquez and Ms. McGuire, Chris was unable to expedite the process. Ongoing miscommunication and installation problems continued to hinder the setup. Even after the approval was received, it was several more weeks before the whole system was finally operational.

Although Edwin at first rationalized the delay as part of the "processing" time, he later told Chris that Jane was slow or she failed to respond to emails or phone calls. Interestingly, Jane said the same of Edwin. Thus, Chris's frequent inquiries of "How's it going? Anything I can do to help move this along?" were answered with "Waiting to hear from Jane" or "Waiting to hear from Edwin." Chris tried to stay in constant communication. His inquires were made by email, phone, and in person at least twice weekly during this 2 month period. Even when access was finally given, Chris was not aware for several days until his next inquiry when Edwin told him that the "approval" process was completed; this was news to Jane as well when Chris contacted her later that day. Chris was pleased that he kept up communication because he might not have learned this for weeks with a more passive approach.

Once the approval was given, it took another 2 weeks for Jane to be given a remote ID and password, which, not surprisingly after the earlier problems, did not work for at least another few weeks after she was given this information. Unfortunately, setting up and using the remote access and connection to the OSI computer required direct and active contact between the information technology staff at both OSI and ASR. By March, it became clear to Chris that Jane and Edwin were not working well together, and in this conflict, they were passive-aggressively deterring progress. Being unable to participate in this process was particularly frustrating to Chris because he could resort only to persistently and continuously inquiring about the progress. Sadly, his email response rate hovered near about one out of five. Jane and Edwin were equally unresponsive to Chris as they were to each other. Frustratingly, when Jane was finally able to access the network and the OSI desktop by remote connection, there was a relatively short time to perform the remote installation.

By the beginning of May, the computer was set up and the software was finally functioning. Chris spent long hours familiarizing himself with the program after a short online tutorial provided by the ASR. At this stage, Chris thought the most difficult part of the project was finally behind him. He trained the staff without major difficulty. The basic use of the software was straightforward as promised by the ASR.

It had simple menus, clear instructions, and touch-screen icons. The trainees included Dr. Smith, several receptionists at the front desk, the clinic nurse practitioner (Liz Brown), and Dr. Smith's long-time clinic nurse (Mary Mulholland). It was decided that only Dr. Smith's patients would participate in the initial implementation because his clinic was relatively small and slow, with at most eight patients in 4 h, twice weekly.

Chris planned to "go live" with the project during the first week in June. He established a protocol to include the computer survey as part of normal clinic workflow (so he thought). The process began before the start of clinic each morning with manual entry of each patient's demographic criteria into Spine Survey. During clinic, the patient was escorted to the Spine Survey computer by a trained staff person who would briefly explain to the patient how to use the program. Staff would direct the patient to the thorough instructions on the introductory screens. The patient would be instructed to read the survey, respond to the questions, and notify the front-desk when finished. Subsequently, the patients would be routed back into the normal clinic workflow for their appointments. Data collected by Spine Survey would be printed at the clinician work area, where Nurse Mary and Dr. Smith could review the information prior to seeing the patients. Additionally, these data were securely stored on the local desktop hard drive with network backup. Finally, Mary or Dr. Smith would enter clinical or operative information using a separate protocol. These entries would be done immediately following clinic or operations, or later in batches as needed. With success of this implementation, the protocol would later be used at Dr. Beck's clinic, which was busier and more frequent than Dr. Smith's. After sufficient data collection, Dr. Beck and Dr. Smith planned to study and publish outcomes of the procedures. Unfortunately, the real world results do not always turn out like the ideal plan.

By the end of the first day of clinic, the process had already gone awry. Chris quickly realized that in order to test the project fairly, he could not rely only on the staff that he had trained. It was evident that Chris would be responsible for much more of the clinic workflow duties than he had planned. Over the next month, he assumed all roles previously assigned to the staff members, who became less cooperative because of the change in their work routine. As previously mentioned, the main responsibilities were inputting patient demographic information at the start of each clinic day and introducing the patient to the system. Operating efficiently, these tasks required approximately 15 min for the day and 2 min for each patient. Chris would enter patient data each morning, wait for the arrival of each patient, and then escort and introduce the patient to the system, as well as respond to technical issues. While none of these tasks were difficult, there was considerable down time between one patient and another, which was highly unproductive for Chris, who did not have work space in the clinic, nor did this seem like relevant research experience.

Early in the implementation, there were a few minor technical difficulties. The software had occasional "bugs" and would crash resulting in the loss of a patient's data. The remote access came in handy in these situations, as Ms. Jeter was able to login and help fix program glitches. However, there were other technical issues with the local network such as setting up a printer for data output and network data backup. Since Edwin was typically slow or non-responsive, these local issues were troublesome.

An important aspect of implementing the survey was choosing information to be collected from each patient. The initial approach was inclusive rather than concise, with the thought that having more data would be better for the research objectives of the project. Therefore, the first few patients were answering a survey that took Chris almost 20 min to complete. He quickly discovered that most patients were much slower, requiring on average about 45 min, and some patients would take over 90 min.

Of course, this seriously affected the normal workflow of the clinic by delaying patients before their appointment in order to collect these data. As there was only one computer, it was impossible to collect data from every patient because an earlier patient was usually still on the computer when the next patient would arrive. The survey was simply too long and the detrimental impact on clinic workflow had an even greater negative impact on staff opinion of the system.

Chris did not realize that each responsibility he took on himself to appease the grievances of the staff was merely a temporary solution. He thought that the clinic staff would slowly respond to his/her enthusiasm and hard work, and each one would eventually accept his/her "appropriate" responsibilities.

Finally, Chris realized that the project was simply not sustainable with his current level of involvement, as he would return to medical school in the fall and could no longer participate as clinic support. Fortunately, Dr. Smith's longtime clinic nurse, Ms. Mulholland, was receptive to taking over Chris's role as the primary steward of the data collection project. She took responsibility for entering demographic data and getting patients to use the survey, by the middle of July. Unfortunately even with a fully integrated work-flow design, the duration of the survey was still a major issue, and generally only one or two patients per clinic were able to participate.

In July, Chris decided to shorten the survey by removing past medical history, social history, family history, and review of systems. Although this decreased the time spent on the survey to less than 20 min for most patients, this still had a notable impact on the clinic workflow. When school began in August, Chris had less time to monitor the functioning of the project. Ms. Mulholland continued to use the system, but small technical issues arose that quickly stirred up the workflow beehive. Mr. Vasquez continued to be unwilling to effectively support the system. Chris was no longer available for immediate troubleshooting. Therefore, the system slowly fell into disuse. It simply became too much trouble for anyone but Ms. Mulholland to operate.

In October, the computer was moved from the office without warning because the office manager decided to reclaim and renovate the office space. The mobile system was taken to a room in the back of the clinic, and data collection stopped completely. With the exception of Ms. Mulholland and Dr. Smith, the office staff felt that the project was a failure. The clinic nurse practitioner, Liz, was particularly averse to success of this project. She had regularly insisted that the system would never work. Ironically, response to her vocal complaints ("too long, too intrusive") and opposition would ultimately lead to a successful implementation.

Cast of characters (in order of appearance)

Name	Position/title	Roles & responsibilities
Chris Ryan	Medical student	Project coordinator and chief implementer
Dr. David Beck	Surgeon	Young faculty, busy with clinic and OR schedule
Dr. Jeffrey Smith	Surgeon; Dept. Chair	Initiation and oversight of project
Fred McCoy	Director of ASR	Consultant to implementation
Edwin Vasquez	Orthopedics LAN manager	Purchase, setup and troubleshooting of hardware; gatekeeper for security and access
Meredith Jeter	Orthopedics office manager	Controls utilization of space
Jane Maguire	ASR IT consultant	Installation and troubleshooting of ASR Spine Survey software
Liz Brown	Orthopedics nurse practitioner	Involved in general clinic functioning
Mary Mullholand	Orthopedics nurse	Managed patient intake and clinic workflow

Questions

1. What mistakes were made by the student in this case? How did these lead to the initial failure of the project?
2. What would you do differently from the start? What solutions would you suggest for the following issues?

   - Physicians
   - Clinic staff
   - Infrastructure/Hardware

3. At the end of this case how might you proceed to re-implement this project and make it successful? (see Epilog)
4. What are the appropriate roles and responsibilities of each of the following characters? Are their expectations reasonable on the basis of this case experience?

   - Student
   - Physicians
   - Clinic staff
   - Support staff (ASR)

5. How could you get buy-in and support from each of the above players for your defined "responsibilities?"
6. Who was the clinic champion of this implementation? Was this role appropriate, and if not who should have had this role?
7. At what point was this project doomed to failure? If this project had not failed completely, could it have been resurrected without a *tabula rasa* approach?
8. How might the changes made in the Epilog improve the functionality and likelihood of successful re-implementation of this system? (How do these changes resolve the problems identified in the implementation of the system?)

Epilog

In December, Chris decided that an overhaul of the program design was necessary for the project to be salvaged. He arranged a meeting at the OSI with Dr. Smith, Dr. Hopkins, an informatics advisor, all of the clinic staff – Ms. Mulholland (RN), Ms. Brown (NP), Mr. Vasquez (IT) – and Fred McCoy, the director of the ASR. At this meeting, the causes of failure in the program's implementation were discussed. The significant problem identified was the impact on clinic workflow. The survey was shortened to include only chief complaint, brief medical history, and outcomes measures (SF-36 and ODI/NDI). Another improvement was to administer the survey at the end of the clinic visit rather than at the outset. The system was also switched to a touch screen tablet PC. In the first iteration, all patients were eligible to participate, whereas in the second implementation, it was decided to include only operative patients, who formed a considerably smaller and therefore more manageable group. The new clinic work-flow protocol was designed to be of very low-impact, requiring little extra effort than the normal process, and considerably less than the original protocol. A final change that was most helpful was assigning a new ASR programmer, Mike Jenkins, to the OSI program. In having all players contribute to the plan there was a greater sense of ownership, which was supported by the mandate for this project from Dr. Smith. Since these changes were made, the project has undergone successful re-implementation and now patients of both surgeons are using the system. The database has over 200 patients recorded in 1 year, which is approximately 75% of the total operative patients seen by Dr. Beck and Dr. Smith. Chris is now completely hands-off, and the system operates with minimal external support from ASR, allowing him to pursue the outcomes "research" aspect of the project.

References

1. Grevitt M, Khazim R, Webb J, Mulholland R, Shepperd J. The short form-36 health survey questionnaire in spine surgery. *J Bone Joint Surg Br*. 1997;79:48-52.
2. Hanscom B, Lurie JD, Homa K, Weinstein JN. Computerized questionnaires and the quality of survey data. *Spine*. 2002;27:1797-1801.
3. Walsh TL, Hanscom B, Lurie JD, Weinstein JN. Is a condition-specific instrument for patients with low back pain/leg symptoms really necessary? The responsiveness of the Oswestry Disability Index, MODEMS, and the SF-36. *Spine*. 2003;28:607-615.

2
A RHIO Struggling to Form: Will it Get Off the Ground?

PAUL ZLOTNIK, DENNY LEE, MIKE MINEAR, and PRASHILA DULLABH

Introduction

As Dr. James Gibbs walked through the parking ramp to his car, he could not get out of his mind the meeting he had just attended. The board of directors of the Mid West RHIO (MWR) had just met, and it was a frustrating meeting for all attendees. The cold and rainy evening was a perfect match to Dr. Gibbs' mood.

Dr. Gibbs had been working to create the capability to share patient clinical data for over 5 years. His passion to improve patient care by ensuring that all clinicians have access to complete data about their patients had in fact fueled the effort to create a regional health information organization (RHIO) before the term was even invented. Certainly, Dr. Gibbs had found a lot of help during the past 5 years, and in the past several years, the group had come tantalizingly close to breaking out of the planning phase of the project towards a launch of the capability to share patient data. But each time something had emerged to slow the effort down or create a roadblock to progress.

After months of work with attorneys and leadership from the key stakeholders, the MWR had finally created a nonprofit corporation that was "owned" by the key stakeholders in the healthcare community. While the new corporate structure was a huge step forward, several of the larger hospital systems in the state seemed to be wavering in their support for the RHIO and were questioning if they should share their patient information with competitors. The technology work group had been working for several years to create a technology plan that could support patient data sharing, but a number of the community physicians felt the plan was too "modernistic" and did not take into account the lack of automation in many physician offices and smaller hospitals. The challenge of funding the MWR had never really been resolved, and although member organizations paid annual dues to keep the organization functioning, these payments were nowhere near the level of funding needed to launch data sharing. Several consumer groups had publicly raised concerns about patient's data being shared to the local newspaper, especially in the light of yet another round of virus attacks embedded in emails and reports of identity thefts.

Worst of all, the leader of the State's Health and Human Services (HHS) agency had recently said in several public forums that he did not support the governance approach of MWR and called for a new form of RHIO based on State control to ensure consumer privacy and regulation compliance. They announced a plan to fund a RHIO planning grant to begin what would amount to a RHIO competing with the MWR.

L. Einbinder et al. (eds.), *Transforming Health Care Through Information:*
Case Studies, Health Informatics, DOI 10.1007/978-1-4419-0269-6_2,
© Springer Science+Business Media, LLC 2010

The seemingly open competition from the State agency had been the most difficult to accept, given the large membership of the MWR throughout the State and the 5 year effort to get the MWR launched.

Perhaps the most frustrating to many of the board members was that the concept of an organization to share patient information made more sense than ever before. The recent disaster from hurricane Katrina had brought home how archaic paper record keeping was in America and how desperately the ability to share patient data on a wide scale was needed. Dr. Gibbs remembered grimly the evening news casts showing how premature infants were transferred out of New Orleans hospitals to other cities, without their parents and without their complete medical records. Evacuees from all across the gulf coast who were waiting for organ donations and those with chronic diseases that required short term medications and follow up struggled to get care in other cities. He remembered reading an article that said that because of the severe flooding, medical records of many of the evacuees were totally destroyed. Even in the Midwest, many miles from New Orleans, a significant number of people had been resettled and many local care providers had seen firsthand the difficulty in recreating medical records from scratch, especially for the elderly or those with chronic diseases.

But the lessons of Katrina had already been learned and relearned by local clinicians for many years. Patients showed up in emergency rooms on a daily basis needing care. A copy of recent history & physicals, current medications, problems lists, recent clinical results, or other basic patient clinical information would be invaluable to ER physicians in providing better and more cost effective care in these settings. Patients constantly move through the healthcare system from primary care physicians to specialists, from clinics to hospitals, and hospitals to home care or nursing homes, but rarely did their clinical information follow along with them.

The lack of shared patient data means that costly clinical tests are repeated and diagnosis takes longer time. The board of the MWR had reviewed the reports from the Center for Information Technology Leadership (CITL). The board felt that CITL's study of the potential economic impacts of information exchange at the community and national level was the most extensive one performed to date. CITL predicted that net savings for HIEI would be $77.8 billion annually, or about 5% of total US healthcare annual expenditures. An element of the CITL study that had made a dramatic impression to board members was that payers – health insurance companies – were by far the most significant economic beneficiaries from HIEI, with an estimated $22 billion per year in savings.[1] Several physicians active in the MWR felt that this analysis of savings rang true and that these national costs savings predictions would translate into real savings to local stakeholders. Given the potential to both improve care and reduce healthcare costs, it seemed that all healthcare stakeholders should strongly support the MWR and help move it forward.

Now it is felt that all the work of so many people for the past 5 years may have been in vain. The board meeting ended with a resolution that unless the funding, privacy, and governance challenges from the State were not resolved within 3 months, the MWR should consider disbanding. Dr. Gibbs knew time could be running out for the MWR and his dream of sharing patient data.

Organizational Background

Early in 2000, Dr. Gibbs had arranged a meeting of key stakeholders to initiate discussions on the formation of the MWR. Prior to that, Dr. Gibbs had engaged with various groups and individuals that he had identified as key stakeholders. His main objectives were to understand current perceptions and to start building support for the creation of the MWR. Dr. Gibbs had consulted with some prominent physicians groups in the area, some local academic and community hospitals, health plans, and payer organizations. His early discussions revealed that there was considerable interest in the creation of the MWR. It was apparent even at that early stage that the motivations of the stakeholders were very different. Dr. Gibbs did not see this as an issue as everyone seemed to be committed to the "common good."

In May 2000, the various stakeholders met for the first time. Present at this meeting were representatives from the key stakeholder group of physicians, both primary care and specialty practices, CIOs from the local academic and community hospitals, and CEOs from the health plan and payer organizations. In addition to these key stakeholders, also present were representatives from professional societies, consumer interest groups, large employers, and various government organizations. Dr. Gibbs was really encouraged by the enthusiastic support demonstrated by the participants and strongly believed that this initiative was going to succeed.

As an immediate next step the membership of the MWR was outlined. On the basis of his prior experience, Dr. Gibbs was acutely aware that in order to ensure success, all parties should have a voice. He therefore became a strong proponent of including professional societies, consumer interest groups, and government organizations as part of the core membership.

As its first objective, the current membership set about identifying the organizational structure. Since RHIOs were relatively new and there were not many industry examples, the membership decided to form an organizational structure that mirrored the various activities that would need to be completed to support the creation of the MWR. On the basis of this, six workgroups were established.

- The steering workgroup
- The provider workgroup
- The technology workgroup
- Data standards and usability workgroup
- The patient privacy and security workgroup
- The public health and outcomes measure workgroup
- Economic outcomes workgroup

The steering workgroup included representatives from all the stakeholders. They were tasked with providing overall leadership and ensuring that the objectives and timelines were established and that each workgroup activity was in concordance with these objectives. The decision making process would be by consensus. The group firmly believed that this approach ensured the greatest buy-in.

On the basis of his discussions with colleagues in other areas and some cursory reading, Dr. Gibbs was aware that building relationships among the various participants in this initiative would be very important. To set the stage for this process, a retreat was arranged where the members of the various workgroups could come together. Dr. Gibbs noticed that although the idea was well received, participation in the retreat was not as high as he would have hoped for. He surmised that this might be related to the timing, and that the enthusiasm that the group displayed was more representative of their commitment.

He was also reminded of the fact that although the group unanimously agreed that the mission was improving patient safety and quality through the effective exchange of information, the motivations of the various stakeholders were very different. For example, the physician groups were largely interested in improving general productivity by having relevant patient information available at the time of care. This would eliminate the need to try and locate patient's records and instead allow the physician access to comprehensive, integrated records that included all facets of a patient's care. The consumer groups were motivated by the possibility of patients now being able to have a more proactive role in their medical management that would hopefully eliminate the need for the numerous office visits. Both the academic and the community hospitals were encouraged by the idea that information exchange would improve efficiency by eliminating the need to track down records from other hospitals, physician practices, and laboratories. There were also other economic motivations of decreasing if not eliminating duplicative testing, enhancing disease management capabilities, and improving claims processing. Not too surprisingly, the payers were by far the most motivated as they would be able to realize benefits on numerous fronts, i.e. better utilization management, increased patient compliance, disease management, and decreased costs associated with duplicative laboratory and radiology tests. Over the course of time, the different motivations of the group would present some of the most challenging aspects of moving the project forward.

As the MWR involved so many stakeholders, the team participated mostly as a virtual team. In order to maintain effective channels of communication, most of the workgroups decided to meet on a monthly basis via conference calls. This approach was augmented by in-person meetings on a quarterly basis. Dr. Gibbs had noted that this approach was not without challenges. Some of these were amplified by the fact that the members came from different cultural backgrounds. It had been years since the inception of this project, and there were still some days when communication among the members seemed to be the biggest challenge.

Just as the coalition was on the verge of bearing the fruits of its efforts, Dr. Gibbs was forced to face the reality that the very tenet on which the organization had been formed was being challenged. He remembered well the early days when the key stakeholders were lobbying for a self governance approach. The culture of the group was very much one of self determination and taking control. Over time, this had become a strong magnet to keep the various stakeholders at the table. With the recent announcements by the leadership of the States' HHS agency that the RHIO should be state governed, Dr. Gibbs had significant doubts as to whether they would overcome this obstacle.

Viewpoints

The barriers to the nationwide establishment of RHIOs as the grassroots of national health information infrastructure are not terribly different from those to the failed creation of CHINs in the early 1990s. However, there is a marked difference in the motivation and leadership that exist in the current era. The stakeholders have broadened to include physicians, hospitals, skilled nursing facilities, home health agencies, laboratories and pharmacies, patients, vendors, payers, and the federal government.[2,3]

Lack of trust is the major barrier at almost all stakeholder levels. Patients have voiced their fears about who will have access to their most sensitive and private health information. They have insisted upon their personal ability to access their records, while insisting upon authorization for sharing, capacity to easily verify who has viewed their records, and emphatically refused to allow employer access of any kind.[4] This reassurance is not only expected from the provider guardians of their healthcare documentation but also from the vendors who are responsible to create the technology to monitor and administer this information. Additionally, the CHINs of the 1990s lacking the internet were forced to use aggregate data repositories, further intensifying distrust and lack of control. Profiling physicians, as well as hospitals, raised the early issues about being competitively disadvantaged.[5] Only by satisfying trust, the industry can potentially hope to avoid the added complexity of "opting in" or "opting out" which could occur at the patient or the provider level.

The entire health-care industry is facing major expenditures for information technology and communication (ITC) equipment during the coming decade. Chief ITC officers are struggling to find the financial capacity to provide electronic medical records (EMRs) to their own organizations,[6,7] let alone additional funds to coordinate external sharing of information. It is estimated that approximately 80–85% of healthcare information on patients exists in small practices. The vast majority of these environments do not have EMRs. Organizations that are ITC operable question whether they should share information with organizations that will not reciprocate.[8] The development of managed care throughout the United States, as well as for-profit hospital networks and insurance underwriters, has compromised the cultural concept of sharing. The current health-care industry thrives on competition and sharing proprietary information is contrary to their bottom line.[8] Further reduction in fee-for-service visits by the expected enhanced quality of care management by the investment and implementation of ITC systems is almost a disincentive for this investment.[6] There are estimates of huge savings from RHIOs, primarily benefiting insurance underwriters, with the establishment of a national integrated delivery network. However, there are neither guarantees that employers will see reductions in premiums nor enhanced funding for healthcare provider's ITC needs. It is yet to be determined whether the pay for performance concept is a big enough incentive to overcome provider's financial hurdles.

Leadership which has been more local in nature needs to change to a national perspective. "Experience teaches us that the private sector does not have sufficient centralized power or the resources to lead an integrated NHII effort."[6] Isolated pockets of regional health information sharing are good demonstrations to justify public–private partnerships as the paradigm of the future. Local, state, and national politics must be put aside to avoid the problems that Dr. Gibbs has experienced. The federal government through funding of research and development has finally created a communications network, "the Internet," that may make data repositories of the early 1990s unnecessary. However, many enterprises may reject a collaborative strategy of "Co-opetition"[2] because they see "their e-health initiatives as a means to competitively distinguish them."[2] The American healthcare industry must look across the Pacific Ocean to Japan to understand that public–private partnerships and co-opetition can benefit competing health-care providers and promote the public good. In response to the Japanese public–private co-opetition in 1975 through 1985 overtaking United States in semiconductor industry, the United States created its own Cooperative Research Act of 1984. As a result of this act the United States regained its leadership in semi conductor research, development, and production. Currently the federal government is leading by example, as well as deterrence, as a result of the implementation of HIPAA. Major hallmarks of HIPAA include the establishment of standards for billing and coding, and penalties for breach in management of personal health information. The establishment of the Office of National Coordinator of Health Information Technology, as well as promotion by the Department of Health and Human Services of a National Health Information Integrated Network (NHIN), is a prime example of leadership at the national level. The only issue that remains is how much leverage must be applied to the providers of health care so that they and the rest of the stakeholders fall in line with the concept of co-opetition. As distasteful as further unfunded mandates have been in the past this may be the necessity for the future.

Information Technology Environment

The creation of the Technology Plan for MWR was a daunting task. While most clinics, pharmacies, and hospitals have desktop computers that connect to the internet, few connect to integrated EMR systems. Like most other RHIO projects across the country, a key factor that exists even today, only around 25% of hospitals have implemented EMR systems while another 40% have contracted or just started their implementations.[9] Most of these systems are not full EMR implementations, typically utilizing just the clinical data repository (CDR), controlled medical vocabulary (CMV), and clinical decision support systems (CDSS) and inference engine. They are very basic and only provide partial solutions, i.e. stage 2 of the 7 stages of a full EMR system.[10] The EMR systems themselves are often different requiring new user training when going from one hospital's system to another.

Even though RHIOs are being rolled out, because of many perceived and real barriers, hospitals and physicians have not readily adopted EMR systems.

> "In general, physicians have known for some time that they will have to go to electronic records," says [C Kerry] Stratford [MD partner in St. George (Utah) Clinic, an eight-member family practice, who automated his practice 2 years ago] "The question is if they go willingly or put it off as long as possible. There is not a universal feeling among physicians that electronic records are the Holy Grail that will solve all of their problems. A lot of fear remains that electronic records will make the practice of medicine harder."[11]

These basic EMR challenges compound the issues that the leaders of the MWR needed to overcome to achieve its goals.

To help Dr. Gibb achieve his dream for the MWR, the technology work group utilized the implementations of an Israeli RHIO[12] built by Clalit Health Services and the guidelines setup by CAL-RHIO for the state of California[13] to build its technology plan and architecture. The key goal for MWR was to allow stakeholders to quickly and safely share patient clinical data, to improve healthcare, and reduce healthcare costs. The first thing that the group did was to insure that there was a clear line of communication among the member organizations. One of the basic tenets of a RHIO is its ability to share data by the use of electronic record and delivery systems. The problem was that many of the clinics and some of the hospitals did not have or only utilized the most basic features of an EMR system. Their primary mode of communication was faxing. The long term plan will be to convert these organizations to electronic medical record systems, but this will take time and money. The bridge gap solution until this is achieved will be procurement and distribution of vendor applications (examples such as DataFax and ProviderLink) which organize and maintain fax images. With hospitals receiving hundreds of faxes a week from other organizations, converting these faxes to indexed images allow any clinician to find the information on an available workstation. More advanced features of virtual fax services include the ability to automate transcription of clinician hand-written notes via optical character recognition (OCR) This information would now be legible and easily added into the patient records of a hospital's EMR.

Having established the capability to communicate and organize clinical summaries between organizations without electronic records, the next issue that needed to be addressed was the how the stakeholders systems could understand each others data. To do this, the workgroup focused on data integration. Working together with the hospitals and clinics within the MWR, the workgroup created a data subcommittee that determined exactly what set of data (e.g. laboratory results, patient notes, x-ray scans, etc.) had to be shared among the MWR participants. The committee determined what standards were followed to insure that the data format from one member organization was the same as that from another. Examples of this include the usage of HL7 for the exchange of administrative data, use of SNOMED to define clinical terminology, and the HL7 RIM to provide a framework for describing clinical data. Additionally it utilized the internet as its communication infrastructure to leverage existing technological infrastructures.

Security and privacy of the patient data followed all of the HIPAA guidelines however there were still many questions that needed resolution by the patient privacy and security workgroup. This workgroup determined the authorization (who is allowed to review the data) and authentication (insuring the person is who s/he says s/he is) models to be implemented. This became more complicated as each hospital has its own authorization/authentication models internally for its interactions with partnering clinics. Therefore, a new set of models was applied on top of the existing hospital/clinic security. But MWRs models did not supersede the existing processes already in place. At the same time, access included a single log on and log off from the systems, which both enhanced usability and minimized security breaches. The plan insured that the data were properly encrypted and that all requests and transfers were logged and monitored, as well as retaining a full audit trail of data and their movements. The committee also determined the type of anti-malware (anti-virus, anti-phishing, firewalls, etc.) utilized and agreed on a common set of standards. This allowed the disparate IT groups within MWR the ability to leverage one another's work and to allow for easier deployment of secure systems.

The next step of the plan was to ascertain the performance and usability of the system. The key here was the ability to quickly access a patient's records. The technology chosen to deploy across MWR needed to respond to all requests for information in under 10 seconds so that medical professionals were not playing a waiting game for vital health information. While the performance/usability workgroup easily established performance metrics, usability was a more difficult issue. The workgroup started by creating concept and use cases that described how participants would utilize the systems within the RHIO. For example a new patient entering into a hospital requiring a record transfer from another hospital as well as a pharmacy electronically sending the patients's prescription history. These scenarios and use cases described how the system would be used. In turn, this insured that users were able to implement, test, and re-implement any part of the system as most medical professionals expected. Service level agreements were created among the participating organizations to clarify the performance and usability expectations within MWR.

Ultimately, the technology work group wanted to build a scalable (ability to handle large volume of data and requests for the data) and extensible (ability to add new features or applications) system. Meeting these goals the system handled the large volume of data and rapid increase in patient record information requests, and easily integrated new participants. The strategy was to build MWR utilizing a federated model instead of a centralized one. As noted above, there were many stakeholder organizations within the MWR, which had already heavily invested in their own EMR systems. No one can afford to give up this investment in order to build a centralized repository of information. As well, the large volume of data spread out among the organizations within the mid-western region would not make it feasible to have only one central repository housing thousands of patients' data. Therefore, MWR had to be able to leverage the large number of existing disparate hospital, clinic, pharmacy, and other participant technology investments. While this made things slightly more complicated for data integration, it insured that the member organizations' own environments were minimally impacted. A centralized model would theoretically achieve a more global view of health information for a community, but the MWRs primary goal was more patient-centric, providing a patient's information irrespective of where it is stored across the network. A federated model achieved the goal of supporting universal data access while leveraging existing stake holder's technology infrastructures and investments.

When the workgroup originally modeled the sharing of data it was relatively easy to insure the accuracy of the patient data. But as more stakeholders were added and data volumes grew it became increasingly difficult to insure the accuracy of the data. For example, if hospital A has "Jon Smith," clinic D has "Jon P Smith," and hospital X has "Jonathan Smith," are they the same person? Accuracy of the data is vital for any RHIO in that mistakes may result in the wrong decision due to incorrect patient history linkage. To resolve this issue, it became clear a master patient index and record locator was needed. This service holds information authorized by the patient about where information can be found but not the actual information itself. This service improved the performance of patient record requests because now the system would only make requests to locations that have the patient's data as opposed to making requests to all participating organizations. This also allows for better security, privacy, and autonomy of participant institutions because it separates the task of identifying where the information is located from the actual releasing and transferring of information to authorized organization that is subject to participating institution regulations.[14]

By creating the above technology plan, the technology work group has created a RHIO architecture that can be leveraged by any State or National Health Information Network. To allow for clear lines of communication, MWR included virtual fax services to treat sheets of paper as portable digital images and utilized standards to allow for clear digital forms of communication. The latest technology is used to insure security and privacy with performance and usability in mind. By using a federated model, we would be able to utilize existing systems and distribute the workload across the entire network. With a master patient index and record locator, we would more accurately and more quickly access patient information and yet keep things more secure. Just as the MWR has planned to leverage the existing infrastructures of the member health organizations, any State or National network will be able to do the same.

Focus of the Case

The Midwest RHIO is experiencing many of the same challenges as faced by many emerging RHIOs across the country. While the vision of the RHIO is powerful, there are many barriers that must be resolved prior to the successful level of data sharing that must be achieved to realize that vision.

Even though the MWR has been incorporated, it has most of the attributes of a virtual organization. What makes any RHIO unique is that to meet the goals of data sharing, it must bring together competitors and organizations of many different types and motivations to accomplish a very difficult goal. There are few success stories on how to effectively share patient data across an entire community. There may be significant legal risk to members who share patient data or decide not to share patient data, or if the data is shared in a flawed manner; the RHIO concept is too new to have a clear sense of the degree of risk absorbed by stakeholders.

Beyond the challenges they have faced to date and the challenges in common with other RHIOs, the MWR is now facing a competition for the future of data sharing in the State. The State HHS agency is intent on creating a RHIO in the State under its control. Even worse, the agency has started a bid process to create a competing RHIO. It is also clear that the State agency is seeking commercial firms to bid for the planning grant. The end result could be a RHIO managed and governed by a commercial for profit firm, or a RHIO governed by the State with a contract to a commercial vendor to manage the operations of the RHIO. In either scenario, the care providers and payers would not have any input and participation in the governance of data sharing in the State.

As it is unlikely that both the MWR and a State sponsored RHIO could exist, only one RHIO is needed. Therefore, the MWR must not only find a way to put its plans into motion but also deal with the challenge from the State agency.

The leaders of the MWR understand that they have reached a critical juncture in their effort. Dr. Gibbs and the other leaders of the RHIO need to create and execute a strategy in the short term to overcome the challenges.

Summary

Achievement of Dr. Gibb's dream of creating the Midwestern RHIO would allow the sharing of important patient data among the clinics, hospitals, pharmacies, and organizations within it. Five years of hard work has created the organizational structure to support the creation and maintenance of MWR with its primary goal to improve patient safety and quality through effective information exchange. With all of the different motivations and viewpoints, the key aspect is to resolve the lack of trust among all of the different stakeholders. Through leadership and expounding the return on investment of the RHIO, the benefits of "co-opetition" and breaking down of the barriers of trust can be achieved. The MWR has designed a technology plan and architecture to insure that health information can be accurately and effectively exchanged. Like many RHIOs, the MWR is at a critical juncture and needs to address both the expected challenges to sharing data and the unexpected challenge from a State agency.

Case Analysis

Politics

The MWR is a nonprofit organization created to achieve clearly defined goals. The leaders of the MWR have been very political, in the sense they have committed themselves to activities that are not necessarily part of their formal job. They have acted in this political manner to accomplish something that had not been done before, i.e. get many organizations to work together and share patient clinical data for the benefit of patients. The State government is totally a political entity, and it is using political means to achieve its goal of controlling the sharing of patient data in the State.

Power

Power is the capacity to influence behavior. The State agency is clearly attempting to use its power to influence the MWR. Certainly, the leadership of the MWR is hoping to use its power, and perhaps create more power, to counter the efforts of the State and bring the vision of the MWR into fruition. Both the leaders of the MWR and the State agency feel it is important to have power and some level of appropriate control over the sharing of patient clinical data in the State.

Stakeholders Satisfaction and Retention

Just as employee satisfaction can be measured and impacted, the stakeholders of the MWR have measurable satisfaction in how the MWR is meeting their needs and goals. The MWR itself was formed to meet a need, the sharing of patient data; as it was not strictly required to share patient data, and care providers got no revenue from sharing, all stakeholders had a more intrinsic reason to share data leading them to support and participate in the forming of the MWR. Each stakeholder's satisfaction will ebb and flow, given the progress the MWR makes towards its goals. It would appear that the efforts of the State agency may negatively impact current stakeholder satisfaction in the MWR.

Strategic Planning

Strategic planning is the process of developing strategies to reach a defined objective. Compared to tactical planning, strategic plans focus on a major goal that often is a dramatic change from the status quo. While the leaders of the MWR must pay attention to many tactical goals, it is critical that they continue to focus on their core strategic goal of the state-wide sharing of patient data. As most strategic goals are, the MWR is trying to achieve something new, difficult, and intensely challenging. The leaders of the MWR have worked hard for 5 years to achieve their strategic vision, and until they reach their goal, they must continue to aggressively pursue their strategic plan, and modify it as needed to deal with new issues and challenges.

Trust

With the delay that is expected from the State's desire for control fabricated on the concern for privacy and regulation compliance, it is essential that the RHIO members embark on some type of small project. Just a small success can demonstrate to the State that what exists is HIPAA compliant and can help maintain momentum. Finding medical homes for emergency department patients or acting as clearing house to see if the uninsured might be eligible for insurance could be considered. Either would be good candidates for funding from health plans or employers.

Change Management

The organizations that are already technology sophisticated need to realize that providing and viewing integrated patient information will be another phase of change. Organizational resistance manifested by structural inertia and resource allocation cannot be minimized. Ability to view all data internally, including information merged from outside sources (labs, x-rays, primary offices, etc.), ideally should be transparent within the existing EMR. Integrating data with needed highlights and/or annotation to identify their external source is no small task. The option of an interim but less seamless process would have information viewed as an "External Data Button Web Page." This would be less burdensome technologically to the organization but require physicians to open a second document which may be less than ideal. Moving forward, organizations can and should place this responsibility upon the vendors of EMRs as the interoperability standards for the CCR (Continuity Care Record) are published.

Leadership

The standards from the public private partnerships and consortiums are more than enough to throw back at the State that another layer of regulations and leadership is unnecessary. The current concept of RHIOs or LHIOs (Local Health Information Organizations) as the leaves on the tree feeding the National Health Information Network (NHIN), that is a much higher node than the State, is our national healthcare system's long term goal.

Culture

From the aspect of organizational culture, MWR is a cosmos of differing characteristics. Some organizations are team oriented while some are innovative and risk taking. Because of this multiplicity, it was important that we all leveraged each other's differences instead of requiring similarity. This understanding of cultures allowed us to achieve a key goal before we were able to exchange health information, the ability to trust each other.

Project Management

Because of the many organizations that had worked together and our multitude of tasks, it was extremely important that the MWR created and utilized a strong project management process to the creation and maintenance of MWR. This would include realistic schedules and plans to implement the planned technology in phases, yet flexible in our implementations. It was especially important that our project management team had built consensus among all of our stakeholders so that we could deliver a framework for specific, measurable, and time-bound goals.

Virtual Teams

In the context of the MWR, the various stakeholders are geographically dispersed. In order that the various working groups get their tasks accomplished, they formed a virtual team that would meet monthly via conference calls. Virtual teams offer a lot of flexibility in how people can come together, but establishing rapport and communication among the various participants is a challenge. Members of the team have to come to know and trust each other in a virtual framework. Building trust is magnified in this context as trust is such a key component of making the RHIO a success.

Communication

Effective communication is the basis of all relationships. There are various different ways in which communication features in the MWR. Firstly the various workgroups had to establish clear means of communication within their respective groups. Secondly they had to establish channels of communication with the Steering Committee. Thirdly the various stakeholders had to communicate back to their various constituents to ensure that they had the support of their member organizations. Because the teams functioned mostly in a virtual context they had to ensure that key information was not lost in translation. Retreats were organized to ensure that there was some opportunity for the Human Moment as described by Hallowell[15].

Motivation

By definition, motivation is the willingness to exert high levels of effort toward organizational goals, conditioned by the efforts' ability to satisfy some individual need. In the MWR there were various stakeholders and the motivations of the various stakeholders were very different. Although everyone was committed to the overall mission of patient safety and quality, many of the stakeholders were motivated by how their respective organizations would benefit from the effective exchange of information. As many of the organizations were competitors, they had to buy-in to the idea of "co-opetition." Working to ensure that individual motivations aligned with those of the organization was one of the key challenges of the MWR.

Groups vs. Teams

A group by definition consists of two or more individuals who interact, are interdependent, and have come together to achieve a particular goal. Some characteristics of groups are that they share information, they generally lack synergy, and they may have a mix of skills that may not be complementary. Teams on the other hand consist of individuals whose efforts result in a performance that is greater than the sum of the individual inputs. Some characteristics of team are that they stimulate creativity, they depend on a collective performance, and they are accountable to both themselves and the team.

On the basis of the criteria highlighted above the MWR is a group. Fundamental to the success of the RHIO is the effective exchange of information among the various stakeholders. The various stakeholders are therefore interdependent as they all have some information that the other organizations could potentially benefit from. The various stakeholders were brought together to pursue the common goal of information exchange. The skills of the various participants are not necessarily complementary and because of their disparate motivations the groups often lacked synergy. By their nature, RHIOs lend themselves to the formation of groups rather than teams.

Question

1. What should Dr. Gibbs focus on next?

References

1. Middleton B. The value of healthcare information exchange and interoperability. Center for Information Technology Leadership Improving Healthcare Value. http://www.citl.org/index.htm.
2. Americans Support Online Personal Health Records; Patient Privacy and Control Over Their Own Information are Crucial to Acceptance. http://www.markle.org/resources/press_center/press_releases/2005/press_release_10112005.php. Accessed 3/18/06.
3. Kaushal R, et al. Functional gaps in attaining a national health information network. *Health Aff*. 2005;24:1281-1289.
4. Overhage M. Indiana Health Information Exchange. http://www.purdue.edu/dp/rche/downloads/ppt/03-22-05_overhage.ppt#306,1; 2005. Accessed 3/18/06.
5. Detmer D. Building the national health information infrastructure for personal health, health care services, public health, and research. *BMC Med Inform Decis Mak*. 2003;3(1). http://www.biomedcentral.com/1472-6947/3/1. Accessed 3/18/06.
6. Rubin R. Community health information movement – where it has been, where it is going. In: O'Carroll PW, ed. *Public Health Informatics and Information Systems*. New York: Springer; 2003.
7. Robinson B. Rhio Resistance. http://www.govhealthit.com/article91429-11-14-05-Print. Accessed 3/18/06.
8. Interviews with health care leaders. 2006 [unpublished].
9. Haskins WK. Hospital CIOs Embrace Electronic Records. http://newsfactor.com, http://news.yahoo.com/s/nf/20060221/bs_nf/417121.
10. Garets D, Davis M. *Electronic Medical Records vs. Electronic Health Records: Yes, There is a Difference*. Chicago, IL: HIMSS Analytics; 2005. http://www.himssanalytics.org/docs/WP_EMR_EHR.pdf.
11. Goedert J. Are RHIOs for real?. *Health Data Manage*. http://www.healthdatamanagement.com/html/current/CurrentIssueStory.cfm?articleId=12877.
12. Blondheim O. RHIO – A Success Story, HIMSS06 Conference – Session 123.
13. CAL RHIO: Framework for Technology Working Group, CAL RHIO. http://www.calrhio.org/workinggroups/technology/meetingmaterials/minutes082505.pdf.
14. Connecting for Health, Markle Foundation. http://www.connectingforhealth.org/.
15. Hallowell EM. The human moment at work. *Harv Bus Rev*. 1999;77(1):58-January/February 1999.

3
A Rough Ride at the Theodore Roosevelt Cancer Center

Karen Albert, Nitika Gupta, Teresa Mason, and Purvi Mehta

Note: *All names of people and places have been fictionalized for confidentiality purposes*

Introduction

Nurse Carolyn Harried walked quickly down the narrow halls of the Theodore Roosevelt Cancer Center (TRCC), rushing to complete her rounds of surgical patients. She could hear the rain pounding at the window, adding to her stress from the busy, difficult shift. Her last patient, Mrs. Surgerized, looked pale, but was sleeping quietly following her radical mastectomy. Nurse Harried glanced at the JP drain inserted at the end of surgery, and noticed there was more drainage since the last check. She jotted down the amount, so that she could record it in the computer's new Intake/Output (I/O) module. Although she had been instructed to use tablet PCs for data entry, she preferred the desktop workstations to the cumbersome tablet setup. She found an open workstation and stared at the blinking Teddy Roosevelt cursor as the log-on process proceeded slowly. The program finally launched, and a couple of screens later she was on the I/O page where she recorded her numbers and printed out the report for Dr. Lerner, the Surgical Fellow on-call for the evening.

Dr. Lerner grabbed a cup of coffee, picked up his patients' charts, and began his review. He was not happy with the new I/O format and wondered why the attending surgeons had not gotten to evaluate this module prior to rollout. He tried to decipher the I/O data, loaded the patient charts onto a cart, and made quick bedside rounds. He noticed that Mrs. Surgerized appeared pale, so he rechecked her I/O numbers which seemed to indicate that there had not been excessive drainage from the JP tube. He noted that a complete blood cell count (CBC) had been ordered for the morning, and he made a mental note to recheck this patient before tomorrow's rounds.

The next morning dawned bright with sunshine, and the newly appointed Project Management Office Head, Maura Reason, gasped when she heard about the incident the previous night. The Chief of Breast Surgery's mastectomy patient had developed a bleeding complication which had almost been missed. The close call was being blamed on the new I/O module which Chief Ezra Powers proclaimed was poorly designed, presented data in an ambiguous fashion, and endangered patients' lives. Dr. Powers was demanding that the module be removed from the system immediately, and he had called an emergency meeting regarding this problem. Maura knew that they should have had the I/O form reviewed by surgeons prior to implementation, but she had

L. Einbinder et al. (eds.), *Transforming Health Care Through Information:*
Case Studies, Health Informatics, DOI 10.1007/978-1-4419-0269-6_3,
© Springer Science+Business Media, LLC 2010

been told that the doctors had refused to do this evaluation. As a result of the confusing form, Mrs. Surgerized's bleeding complication was not recognized quickly. Fortunately, the patient's morning CBC had alerted staff to the problem, so she had been rushed back into surgery and was then resting comfortably.

"At least the rest of the new nursing system implementation has gone well," Maura thought. Just then, the phone rang and Lotta Douts Associate Director of Nursing, demanded, "We need to talk about the tablet PCs my nurses are being asked to use!" Maura took a Tylenol™ capsule from her drawer. "This is going to be one of those days..." she mused.

Organizational History/Background

TRCC is a National Cancer Institute-designated comprehensive cancer center formed in 1968 by the union of the Benjamin Rush Research Institute and the Meadowbrook Cancer Hospital. It is one of a small group of elite institutions combining cutting-edge research with oncology-focused patient care. Focusing on small a core mission of conquering cancer through prevention, treatment, and research, the Center has grown since its founding, expanding from a few hundred personnel to more than 2,000 FTE. Its research component is known for award winning work (three Nobel Prizes, two Lasker Awards), and its clinical care is highly rated on local and national hospital surveys. The nursing department was one of the first in the country to be awarded Magnet status, boosting the overall reputation of the hospital's patient care and helping improve nurse recruitment and retention. The Center is located within the city limits of a large metropolitan area which is nationally known for outstanding healthcare, creating an extremely competitive environment for cancer treatment facilities. TRCC staff are proud of their long and distinguished history of research and high-quality clinical practice. The shared goal of "conquering cancer through prevention, treatment, and research" brings staff a sense of meaning and importance to their work, which can be motivational even under trying circumstances. To insure continued communication between researchers and clinicians, long-standing traditions, such as daily tea and cake in the late afternoon, continue even today. The somewhat conservative organizational culture emphasizes preservation of the status quo, although the competitive healthcare environment stimulates pursuit of the most current medical practices and advanced technologies. However, two out of three VPs interviewed indicate that the institution is generally resistant to change. The Center's organizational structure is substantially a top-down machine bureaucracy led by a Board of Directors, President, and Chief Operating Officer (COO), as well as numerous Vice Presidents with associated formal reporting structures. In addition, the medical staff is organized as a professional bureaucracy, with all doctors employed by the Center.

IT Structure

Earlier, computing at the Center was organized around a feudal-like structure, with distinctively separate IT operations for research, medical/administration, and radiation oncology, a single department with a high patient census and a strong, nationally known leader. This model eventually became problematic, due to a lack of uniformity of software, hardware, and technical support, and more importantly, overall inconsistency in the development of a unified vision for future information technology planning. As a result of several large strategic planning retreats and sessions involving middle and upper management, a decision was made to hire a Chief Information Officer (CIO) to unify information science and technology (IS&T) institution-wide. In 2002, the CIO was recruited and hired as the first and only external Vice President ever appointed at the Center. This is reflective of the somewhat change-resistant, insular nature of the organizational culture at TRCC.

The new CIO was charged not only with consolidating the three computer center "fiefdoms" into one department, but also with moving the Center closer to implementation of more cutting-edge clinical and research computing systems. The main focus of the IS&T department's current strategic plan is to close the clinical loop through continued improvement of the institution's electronic medical records, thereby fostering the business drivers of patient safety, regulatory compliance, and efficiency. Structurally and politically, the IS&T Department has operated as a centralized monarchy under the CIO's leadership; however, there are signs of movement toward more of a federalism-type model of political leadership and a decentralized or matrix-type organizational structure.[1]

Focus of the Case

The focus of this case is TRCC's nursing documentation system, which was implemented in 2006 as Phase II of the organization's evolution toward a total electronic health record (EHR). The history leading up to this implementation is important in understanding the major issues of the case, which demonstrate the interplay of organizational and technical factors known to strongly influence the outcomes of informatics projects.[2,3]

Following his arrival in 2002, CIO Maxwell Sharpe, MD, was charged with developing an overall strategy for moving forward with clinical system implementations. Sharpe inherited some outside consultants whom he charged with creating a comprehensive clinical systems strategy. Based on this work as well as input from TRCC staff planning retreats, the CIO drew up a 5-year strategy for moving to a complete EHR including computerized physician order entry (CPOE). At the time, TRCC clinicians were accustomed to using a homegrown legacy clinical records information system (CRIS), which was mainly designed for viewing laboratory, radiology, and dictated reports. CRIS was user-friendly and well liked by doctors, but it had to be phased out because it was not HIPAA-compliant and had no capability for audit trails. The CIO and IT leadership knew that a more comprehensive system was needed, which would include functions such as scheduling, CPOE, and the ability to build a patient database.

Clinical System Vendor Selection

In 2002, a multidisciplinary group of 40 TRCC staff embarked on a 6-month planning process to develop a CRIS replacement strategy. This committee recommended a "best of cluster" approach, which would implement groupings of clinical applications around strong vendor products in appropriate areas.[4] To select a central EHR vendor, a team of 12, including doctors, nurses, administrators, and other clinical staff, did an exhaustive search of the marketplace, wrote an RFP, reviewed proposals and demonstrations, and narrowed the field to two major vendors, Morgan and Niles (its Visionex product). Following a site visit to a cancer center using Morgan, the COO provided the CIO with feedback which stimulated the group to select Niles as the preferred vendor on the basis of geographic proximity, financial incentives, and a promise to customize and deliver an oncology module. According to several team members, the selection of the Niles Visionex system represented a reversal of the group's original choice (Morgan), but was made after top administrators, including the CIO, advocated for Niles. Vendor options were limited, as companies with more viable systems would not bid on the contract. Each of the two finalists had drawbacks. Morgan references were weak, while Visionex was new and untested. Everyone hoped Niles would live up to the promise it appeared to have. Several team members felt that this top-down style of decision making dampened their enthusiasm and buy-in for the project. It does appear to contradict informatics change management principles which emphasize the importance of fostering stakeholder involvement and empowerment.[5]

Phase I Implementation: User Resistance and Impact on Phase II

The main clinical application was rolled out in stages – with Phase I, Visionex Clinical Access, implemented in 2004; and the Clinical Documentation System (CDS-Phase II) following 2 years later. Phase I's move from the popular CRIS application to an entirely new system for viewing results, physician notes, etc. represented a significant organizational change for the Center's clinical staff and set the stage for challenges associated with the nursing documentation phase that followed.

Administrative leaders acknowledge there was some clinician resistance to the initial Visionex implementation. These attitudes are supported by survey data that compare user views of CRIS (baseline information) with opinions of Visionex (Phase I) between 2004 and 2005. Results show that while average scores on Visionex user satisfaction questions are worse than the baseline data on CRIS, the differential is not huge; later surveys show improvement. Some respondents' narrative comments demonstrate strong negativity, perhaps reflecting that the limited number of survey questions did not address the full range of user reactions.

Initial survey comments reflect a common form of clinician resistance involving unfavorable comparisons with the prior system[6]:

- CRIS was so much easier to use and accessing reports was so much faster.
- Visionex is more time-consuming than CRIS.

Other comments reflect concerns about "perceived low personal benefits" and "fear of wasted time"[6] due to system-related issues:

- Visionex is still unwieldy and requires extra steps. It is inefficient. Much of the old data is still in CRIS. Modify or REPLACE!!!
- It is not easy and takes too long to scroll back to older reports.

Clinical system implementations can trigger negative emotions and resentment when the system seems to interfere with reaching clinical goals.[7] The following reflect this type of frustration:

- Get a new system WHATEVER the cost.
- It's a real lousy system!
- Visionex is a nonintuitive, bulky, clumsy system with a user interface designed by a sadist...
- Visionex so far is a disaster...

A year after the Visionex Clinical Access implementation, survey responses and project leaders indicated improvement in user acceptance. In addition, in-house information technology (IT) staff developed patches and enhancements to the system, including a streamlined single sign-on process and easy-to-use links to other information systems – such as pharmacy and radiology. In spite of these improvements, some physicians still note system deficiencies, such as general slowness, a small onscreen window, and a less than optimal user interface. In addition, unresolved Phase I issues appear to have affected aspects of the Phase II project.

A universally accepted antecedent of successful clinical system implementations is clinician involvement in the relevant change processes.[8-11] This includes seeking input at the earliest stages and throughout the process.[5] The Visionex Phase II Intake/Output (I/O) incident could likely have been avoided had surgeons reviewed this module before it was implemented. Reasons behind the lack of involvement of MDs in the I/O module review are perceived differently by each of the groups involved – but negativity about Visionex may have played a role.

According to surgeon, Dr. Raleigh Troups, since physicians' complaints about Visionex Phase I had not been fully addressed, the medical staff gave up on providing input. Dr. N. Too Teck, medical oncologist and Medical Director, Ambulatory Care, said: "*We were not asked to participate.*" The CIO and other administrators said some doctors reviewed the module, but surgeons, in particular, declined to follow through, indicating that the CDS was primarily for nurses. Doctors did rely on the intake/output information entered by nurses, and shortly after CDS implementation, data from the module was recognized as inadequate and ambiguous. The module was brought down after it failed to provide the information needed to properly assess one patient's postoperative bleeding problem. According to Dr. Troups, some physicians believe it took this patient safety issue for action on the clinical system to be taken, whereas prior complaints about system deficiencies had not been fully addressed. However, Dr. Troups joined the TRCC staff several years after the Phase I implementation; his past experience with a fully functional EHR may have elevated his expectations, prompting him to view Visionex more negatively.

It is also notable that one of the Center's surgical oncology fellows, Dr. O.K. Nugai, has a more positive take on Visionex, saying, "*All systems have problems. Visionex is fairly user-friendly and I like the fact that I can access a patient's past history even back to the 90s.*" But Drs. Troups and Teck agree that communication between TRCC physicians and the administration could be better. Dr. Troups indicates that MDs still question why the administration "*sticks with Visionex despite its obvious deficits and the many complaints about it.*" He notes that the monthly lunchtime user group meetings are inconvenient for most doctors, making it difficult for some to communicate their concerns. He is pleased that he has been asked to form a Physicians' Advisory Committee, and he has recruited nearly a full contingent of members representing all medical departments. He hopes this will bring more MDs back into the process and restore their trust, since as he says: "*There's no way to get to Order Entry without improving this situation.*" Drs. Sharpe and Teck fully support Dr. Troups' leadership of this group, acknowledging that as part of the Center administration, neither of them could have successfully filled this role. In addition, several other staff committees, such as CPEST (Clinical Projects Executive Steering Team) and SLUG (System Leads User Group), provide valuable project oversight and serve as venues for some user involvement.

Nursing Documentation – Use of Consultants and Goals/Objectives

The CDS (Visionex Phase II) was designed to allow nurses and other allied health professionals to record vital signs: pain, fatigue, and other assessments; Intake/Output (I/O); and allergy data at the patient's bedside via tablet PCs with a computer pen input device. The system was deployed in both inpatient and outpatient areas after a lengthy planning and design period led initially by two groups of outside consultants and later by an in-house project management team. While CIO Max Sharpe has strong praise for the consultants' work, current project leaders fault them for slowing the process and having difficulties coordinating with each other. As outsiders, consultants can provide an objective perspective and function as effective change agents, although they can be disadvantaged by having weaker buy-in and less complete knowledge of institutional history and culture.[12] PMO head, Maura Reason, indicates that prolongation of the project led to some loss of enthusiasm downstream.

It is also not clear that motivational goals were uniformly articulated and communicated by project leaders throughout the planning and implementation process. The Phase II charter identifies the project's main objective as support for the organization's evolution toward an Electronic Medical Record, an overarching message that is clearly communicated by organizational and project leaders. However, there are other benefits of computerized nursing documentation systems that could serve as greater incentives for building user buy-in. These include the potential to achieve time efficiencies,[8,13,14] as well as resolve quality issues reportedly associated with paper-based nursing documentation.[15,16] These factors and others such as decreased medication errors, improved nurse–physician cooperation,[17] and assistance with nursing care planning,[18] could motivate nurses toward greater acceptance of electronic solutions. TRCCs additional charter objectives of improved access to the medical chart, support for clinician workflow, optimization of clinician productivity, and delivery of safe patient care are also potentially motivational.

Nurses' overall perceptions of effective use of their time can have a significant impact on the success of a documentation system implementation.[19] Time efficiency was cited as a potential incentive by CDS project manager, Lida Team, but this benefit is apparently not currently being realized and is a problem in other clinical documentation implementations as well.[20] Only a relatively small portion of TRCC's full nursing documentation process is live on the system, and alert triggers have not yet been activated to address patient safety issues and provide more motivational attainment of original charter goals. As Lida Team says, *"Having workflows and alerting features of CDS at go live would motivate staff because this should improve patient care. These are future enhancements hoped for by clinical staff."*

Nursing Documentation – Teams, Training, and Implementation Support

Teams of representative users were used extensively in the planning for CDS implementation. Several committees, such as GAD (Group Application Design) and CPEST were formed to aid in this process. Executive sponsors, including several VPs, the CIO, and Chief Technology Officer (CTO), met regularly with the project team to provide management involvement and support. According to Lida Team, the GAD group of 40 nurses was large and diverse, routinely meeting to make design decisions. But the group suffered from inconsistent leadership and excessive size, which tended to slow project movement overall. GAD was eventually replaced by a smaller committee to help streamline the decision making process.

Pre-implementation communication and training were well managed, with hands-on mandatory end-user sessions provided to all nurses. Fifteen nurses conducted the 2-hr classes, and computer-based training (CBT) modules were developed to provide an alternative learning format. Effective utilization of this multimedia-type of training has been shown to enhance overall user acceptance of such systems.[18] TRCC nurse educators specially trained a number of super-users, and two nurse champions now serve as the CDS project leaders. There was a special 24/7 telephone support hotline and rotating support staff initially, while the institutional Help Desk handles ongoing issues.

Postimplementation Issues

In spite of the in-depth training and support provided for nurses on the software and associated tablet PCs, many still do not use the system for bedside data recording. Nurses and project leaders acknowledge the continued practice of dual documentation, a known issue associated with some nursing systems.[21,22] While Center nurses are generally using the system to chart vital signs and allergies, managers note the continuing struggles to take full advantage of electronic documentation, as below:

Cheri Leader, Executive Director of Nursing: "*Nurses are not really doing too much with it at this time... We think that with V4 [next version], they will start doing much more clinical documentation.*"

Lotta Douts, Associate Director of Nursing: "*The CDS system did not decrease the workload of the nurses because even today half of the documentation is done on paper. It is a problem putting some information in the computer, so sometimes nurses just ignore it. They just do it on paper.*"

Donna Backer, Nursing Systems Analyst: "*... the nurses at the moment are jotting down the vitals, allergies, etc. on a piece of paper and then going to the nurse's station to input the data on the computer there. The tablet PCs are still not being used in front of the patient.*"

These same nurses are critical of the Visionex poor response rate and cumbersome interface:

Cheri Leader: "*It is so slow... it can make you nuts sometimes.*"

Lotta Douts: "*The system is not very user friendly. ...there are a lot of screens you have to work through.*"

The tablet PCs seemed like an ideal way to provide adequate computer access for nursing staff. Unfortunately, the computer pen input devices and tablet set-ups overall were not well accepted in inpatient areas at TRCC. Even tablets placed atop COWs (carts on wheels) are too large to fit comfortably into small patient rooms. As a further usage hurdle, inpatient area tablets are housed in locked metal wall units with unwieldy doors requiring significant pressure to keep them in the open position while keyboarding. A much better design is available in outpatient areas where a wall mounted tablet sits uncased above a shelf holding a full-sized keyboard. Keyboards were added to address problems with the original pen inputting device. To help address these types of issues, one study recommends usability assessments prior to implementation to solicit suggestions from nurse users regarding optimal hardware configurations.[21]

The advanced average age (over 45) of TRCC nurses and their general lack of computer skills add to these problems, which could possibly have been anticipated with more direct observation and greater nursing input into the workflow redesign process.[23] Age and lack of computer skills have been shown to correlate with less favorable attitudes and lower adoption of computer-based nursing documentation.[18,21] Acceptance of these systems can be influenced by nurse self-confidence in computer use. In addition, computer system "fit" is important; in other words, how well the new system functions to support the true nursing documentation tasks.[16,20] TRCC project leader, Anna Liza Lott, acknowledged the need to better analyze pre-implementation workflow and then work with users to assess the new processes requiring post-implementation. PMO Manager, Maura Reason, indicates that this type of analysis is routinely done at the Center; nonetheless, the resulting CDS adoption problems appear related to workflow analysis deficiencies.

TRCC Evaluation and Project Closing Document

A formal evaluation of the Phase II implementation has not been done, although both Lida Team and Shirley Overseer, VP, Hospital Services, agree this would be beneficial. Maura Reason acknowledges that end users would need to be interviewed or surveyed to assess their opinions of the system. The project's draft closing document fails to mention the problems with dual documentation and the tablet PCs. However, Lida Team reports that the final completed charter document includes two very important lessons learned, that is:

1. Have one leader oversee planning sessions.
2. MDs should be involved in the design process.

The second lesson was already applied in developing two later modules of the CDS; namely, "pulse oximetry" and "arterial blood gases." The CIO indicates that physician input was critical to the successful implementation of these two online report forms.

Unique Needs of a Cancer Center System

Several stakeholders indicated that there are special challenges faced by cancer centers in implementing a clinical system, which is why the development of a Visionex oncology module was so appealing during the vendor selection process. Oncology practice is outpatient-focused and schedule-dependent due to the multitude of testing, follow-up appointments, and therapies required, driving the need for clinical system to handle this complicated and coordinated scheduling process. Maura Reason says that cancer patients are treated on an ongoing, possibly lifetime basis, and that data from past visits must be available to doctors. In addition, many cancer patients are on clinical trials, and that information should also be incorporated into the EHR. These functions have not been addressed by Visionex, a deficit that most Center leaders acknowledge with some disappointment.

Stakeholders' Points of View – Where Do We Go from Here?

CIO Max Sharpe says there are no other clinical systems available that can fully address the special needs of a cancer center, especially in the outpatient setting. He acknowledges having problems with both phases of the Visionex implementation and gives Phase I a grade of "C," and Phase II a "B." However, he proudly notes that over 25 clinical systems were successfully launched in the 5 years since he arrived at TRCC, and out of all of these implementations, the problematic I/O module was the only portion of any system that had to be taken down. He regrets that when the Niles selection was made, there was no viable structure for involving more stakeholders in the decision, since this could have prevented the pockets of negativism that persist today. He also regrets being 2 years behind schedule for CPOE, and acknowledges the need to be more proactive in soliciting user involvement.

Shirley Overseer says that the nurses' participation in Phase II planning was pretty heavy, and they are satisfied with the system. She believes that the next version of Visionex (V4) will be more tailored to physician needs and have a new, more acceptable, I/O module. She thinks that vendor systems have their limitations, and physician involvement is very necessary. She would embrace user satisfaction surveys being done after this new version is implemented.

Cheri Leader believes they should have involved physicians at ground zero. There was an attempt, but she says the administration should have been much more aggressive and insistent about engaging their participation. She thinks that CIO Max Sharpe has made a huge difference overall and that Dr. Raleigh Troups is working hard to pull everyone together.

Lotta Douts says that one of her major concerns is system speed. She also notes that nurses' lack of computer skills including the ability to surf the Web and using email can add to system usage problems overall.

Donna Backer is pleased that nurses were so heavily involved in the decision-making process connected with the CDS implementation. She, along with another nurse analyst, are happy to serve as champions for the new system.

Abel Fix, Technology Support & Development Pharmacist, believes that Niles Visionex is basically "vaporware," and it needs lots of patches. He believes that the vendor selection process was not handled well and although all hoped Niles would be better than expected, their concerns about the system have proven to be justified. But he says everyone will keep trying to make things better.

Dr. N. Too Teck indicates that TRCC is a conservative organization, so change is difficult. He says that the administration and physicians do not necessarily agree on things, such as Visionex. He blames the I/O debacle on the consultants who "*never involved the physicians in anything they were doing.*" But, he notes that now there is a committee (which he chairs) with broad representation to review clinical systems and projects. He believes that CPOE will happen in a few years, and that doctors will be forced to use it. He says: "*They won't have a choice in the matter.*" But he indicates that they are spreading the word about CPOE and are attempting to get everyone involved.

Anna Liza Lott thinks there is a need to spend more time with users to better address workflow and process changes which contributed to problems with the CDS implementation.

Maura Reason and Lida Team acknowledge that their takeover of the leadership of Visionex Phase II from the outside consultants got the project moving and on track.

Maura's headache over the I/O debacle has subsided, but she and the other project leaders still wonder how to address the problems with tablet PCs, double charting, and lack of enthusiasm for the system overall. At times, Maura cringes when she recalls that following the Phase I implementation, doctors were repeating the phrase: "Send Niles running for miles." She certainly does not wish to return to that phase! Maura hopes that the new Physicians' Advisory Group will be able to rally more doctor support for Visionex and future implementations such as CPOE, and she is counting on the hiring of a physician informaticist to champion the cause of the MDs.

Question

The basic question that remains is:

1. What can be done to correct problems with the current CDS and ensure success of future Center implementations like CPOE?

Analysis of Issues and Recommendations

The main issues associated with the current CDS and impacting the future implementations are:

1. Communication gaps and less than optimal user satisfaction, empowerment, and involvement.
2. Tendency toward a top-down style of leadership and decision making.
3. Lack of a clear, unified vision and consistently communicated motivational goals.
4. Workflow redesign problems impacting the usage of the CDS as intended.
5. Technical deficits of Visionex in general.
6. Managing resistance to change.

Communication Gaps – User Satisfaction Issues

Difficulties gaining user satisfaction and acceptance for Visionex Phase I impacted Visionex Phase II, most visibly with the failure of the I/O module, primarily due to lack of participation by surgeons in the system review process. Differing points of view persist on this issue and on Visionex acceptability in general, indicating some communication gaps between institutional users and leaders. There are currently no true MD champions of the Niles clinical system, although there are several effective nurse systems analysts who serve in this role. Virtually, all TRCC stakeholders interviewed agree that more physician involvement and empowerment are essential for going forward.

There are also nursing acceptance issues with Visionex Phase II, evidenced by continuing dual documentation practices, the underutilization of tablet PCs, and complaints from nurse leaders about system deficiencies. No surveys have been done on this phase to assess overall user satisfaction and the extent of the problems encountered, although several leaders indicate that surveys will be done following implementation of the next version of Visionex. Nursing involvement was strong throughout the CDS module development process.

Finally, it is notable that original outside consulting groups did not communicate well with each other and were somewhat resented by Center staff, although the CIO was happy with the work of the consultants and says they were a convenient target for TRCC staff complaints about the clinical system.

Recommendations

- Heighten physician involvement and empowerment

  - Continue with formation of a Physicians' Advisory Group to allow user input and a means for communicating with administration about current and future issues pertaining to system implementations. This process could help increase MD responsibility, empowerment, and motivation,[24] to address persistent MD negativity.
  - Hire a physician informaticist to serve as an MD champion or resource for developing internal physician advocates who understand systems to be implemented.[11] With impetus from clinical staff, physicians are likely to adapt to system changes more quickly and fully.[25]
  - Ensure that all relevant end users are represented in review and verification of online CDS forms prior to implementation.

- Establish feedback mechanisms involving nurses and doctors

  - Survey or interview nurses to obtain user feedback, providing a means for continuous improvement. Results of these surveys should be shared with the staff and used to determine nurses' specific needs and preferences for system modifications.[21]
  - Change user feedback meetings from lunch hour to another time more convenient for clinical staff – or vary meeting times to encourage broader attendance.

- Additional communications steps:

  - Hold regular meetings of a team comprised of the PM, nurse champions, physician and surgeon champions, IT and Niles representatives.
  - Over-communication early in the process and throughout is an important prerequisite to success.[26,27] Use multiple information channels, and involve top and middle management in listening to users' concerns to ensure that staff perceive that they are being heard.[26]
  - Any future use of outside consultants should be carefully planned with specific time-limited objectives well defined[28] and emphasizing bidirectional communication with in-house staff.

Top-Down Leadership and Decision-Making

Top-down leadership and decision-making style have caused problems in several areas of this case. The main vendor selection process, while initially participative, was ultimately controlled by top management, and more importantly, perceived by some as resulting in an imposed decision. The implementation of tablet PCs and rollout of the I/O module model also reflect this tendency toward making decisions without full participation of relevant user groups. In addition, CPOE implementation is being viewed – at least by one Center leader – as a system that doctors will be "forced" to use, although communication with end users about this is also recognized as important.

Recommendations

- Use more participative decision making in selecting systems and fine-tuning capabilities. Grass roots involvement helps generate commitment,[29] and building ownership early can overcome resistance caused by technical deficits.[24] TRCC needs to continue moving toward this type of decision making, as it has been doing with formation of committees like CPEST.
- Varied user groups, including end users and top management, should be represented as part of the decision-making process.
- Shift IS&T from the current centralized (monarchy) model, in which most power resides with the CIO, toward more decentralization and a federalism-type political model in which *"people with different interests work out... a collective purpose and means for achieving it."*[1]
- Modify the "top-down" attitude of administration, since this type of approach can be problematic in clinical system implementations, especially CPOE.[26] Forcing CPOE on the users could be counterproductive, whereas a more collaborative approach is generally more successful.[25]

Lack of a Unified Vision and Consistently Communicated Motivational Goals

The overarching vision of moving to an EHR at TRCC aligns with the organization's strategic plan, but communication of this vision and supporting goals have appeared weak at times. When asked about their goals for the CDS, the CIO, VP for Ambulatory Care, and VP for Nursing Care at TRCC had disparate answers. TRCCs Phase II charter identified some potentially motivational project objectives which were not uniformly mentioned in nursing and project leader interviews. With all of the Visionex deficiencies, clear, inspiring goals are especially important, since as Lorenzi and Riley say: "Motivated, enthused people can make a relatively weak system work."[6]

Recommendations

- Ensure that staff at all organizational levels, from top management to end users understand the organization's strategic goals,[30] as well as the overall vision and supporting objectives for clinical system implementations. TRCC leadership need to

agree on and frequently communicate a clear vision and more motivational goals for CDS, such as time efficiency, improved documentation quality, and patient safety.
- Clearly communicating that CDS objectives align with the organizational goal of working toward a Electronic Medical Record would encourage stakeholder buy-in and support for new system implementations.[30]

Workflow Redesign and Training Issues Associated with the CDS

The manner in which an electronic clinical application integrates into existing environments and workflow is critical to its success. The TRCC nursing staff expected the electronic CDS to improve their efficiency, providing more time for patient care. This was not the case, as there is still dual documentation and under utilization of the tablet PCs for recording information at the patient's bedside. Tablet PC usage problems are most pronounced in the outpatient areas.

Interviews with the nursing staff reveal some nurses having a general discomfort with computers,[31] including even the basic use of internet and email. The advanced average age of Center nurses means that many lack significant computer experience and confidence.

Recommendations

- Analyze the existing workflow and implement systems accordingly. Modify and streamline problematic areas before system rollout. The regular documentation processes should be carefully examined and analyzed with regard to computer support.[32]
- Ensure that the nursing staff is involved throughout the analysis to create possible solutions and to build ownership in the solution.[33] Use a combination of surveys, interviews, and observation to gain an understanding of nurses' needs, preferences, and practices in connection with the current system and any future versions implemented.[21,23]
- Thoroughly test users on both software and hardware components. Evaluate a possible change in hardware that would make nursing documentation an easier task.
- Addressing human–computer interaction (HCI) challenges associated with clinical information systems is paramount.[34] HCI challenges encountered at TRCC (use of the tablet PCs) could possibly be improved by enlisting the aid of external HCI consultants.
- Since formal computer training can alleviate computer discomfort and facilitate clinical systems use,[18,19,21] institute hands-on computer training sessions for nurses, starting with general computer skills, basic internet, and email usage, and progressing to the use of Visionex.
- Institute a recognition or reward system for successful nurse users.

Technical Issues with Visionex

Visionex has been criticized for its lack of user friendliness, and clinical staff have complained that the system is slow and requires navigating through multiple screens before locating necessary information. There has been general disappointment because the promised oncology module has not been developed, and Niles has not addressed EHR needs unique to a cancer center with a strong outpatient focus and intricate patient scheduling.

Recommendations

- Consider seeking a separate commercial system incorporating ambulatory care and scheduling function needs specific to a cancer center.
- Set up a working committee to assess the special system needs of the institution and to work with Niles to address these.
- Management should try and show small but frequent implementation successes to the staff to gain their confidence and restore credibility. Dr. Raleigh Troups is already planning to use this technique with his Physicians' Advisory Board.
- Visit other cancer centers to gain ideas on how they implement EHRs and CPOE.[35,36]

Managing Resistance to Change

TRCC doctors and nurses exhibited some of the typical resistance to changes imposed by new clinical system implementations. Physicians' negative reactions and desire to return to CRIS may have come from perceived low personal benefits, fear of wasted time or forced system routines,[6] and insufficient involvement in the change process.[5] Overt resistance occurred over the I/O module and was dealt with quickly; however, some subtle or deferred resistance remains which could be more difficult to address over time.[12]

Some nurses have resisted using the CDS as originally intended. Recommended tactics for overcoming resistance to change can improve adaptation to and acceptance of system implementations.[6,12] Although TRCC has followed many organizational change principles, some problem areas remain.

Recommendations

- Determine system benefits and communicate to users the compelling reasons for the change.
- Attack negativity in the general institutional climate using sound organizational development techniques and embracing openness, trust, respect, and collaboration.
- Recruit system champions – respected clinical staff members, who accept change and have strong self-confidence and high tolerance for risk.
- Build staff ownership in the system via user involvement, participation and communication.
- Implement rapidly to avoid losing momentum and enthusiasm.[6,12]
- Manage user expectations realistically, by clearly and frequently articulating and communicating system limitations.[37]
- Provide timely and high-quality training and extensive system support.[6]

Conclusion

TRCC has done many things right. The organizational culture tends toward conservatism and resistance to change, although the top administration has shown patience and understanding with the inevitable delays and difficulties associated with clinical system implementations. Also to its credit, the Center boldly hired a well-respected

CIO from outside the organization and embarked on drastically changing the IT structure as well as implementing a host of new clinical systems, most of which have been successfully launched within a relatively short period of time. The problems associated with this case demonstrate the strong interrelationship of technical and organizational issues. In implementing the nursing documentation system, Center IS&T leadership recognized the importance of organizational factors, making good use of teams to solicit user input and establishing in-depth training and support for the new system. A number of problems occurred due to unrecognized system defects caused by lack of surgeon involvement, weaknesses in hardware usability assessment, and some deficits in overall workflow analysis. Pockets of user negativity toward the clinical system remain, fostering some "we/they" divisiveness between the administration and clinical staff. TRCC leaders are taking steps, such as implementing a Physician's Advisory Group and recruiting a physician informaticist, to address these problems. Technical issues with the current commercial system continue, although the latest version of Visionex may resolve many of these problems. Organizational factors will remain important to the success of future implementations.

TRCC has in its favor a strong shared mission of "conquering cancer through prevention, treatment and research," which inspires staff to persevere under trying circumstances, encouraging the pursuit of strategies to make things work. While the Center has had somewhat of a "rough ride" with aspects of its nursing documentation system, there is reason to remain optimistic, because action is being taken, including some of what is recommended here, to ameliorate current problems and ensure success with future clinical system implementations.

Question

1. What should the CIO do? What sequence of steps would you recommend?

References

1. Lorenzi NM, Riley RT. Understanding and analyzing organizational structures. In: Lorenzi NM, Riley RT, eds. *Managing Technological Change*. New York: Springer; 2004.
2. Aarts J, Doorewaard H, Berg M. Understanding implementation: the case of a computerized physician order entry system in a large Dutch university medical center. *J Am Med Inform Assoc*. 2004;11(3):207-216.
3. Berg M. Implementing information systems in health care organizations: myths and challenges. *Int J Med Inform*. 2001;64(2-3):143-156.
4. Hagland M. Interoperability conundrum: EMR implementation options go beyond core vendor and best of breed. *Healthc Inform*. 2005;22(5):28-30, 32, 34.
5. Lorenzi NM, Riley RT, Blyth AJ, Southon G, Dixon BJ. Antecedents of the people and organizational aspects of medical informatics: review of the literature. *J Am Med Inform Assoc*. 1997;4(2):79-93.
6. Lorenzi NM, Riley RT. Gaining physician acceptance. In: Lorenzi NM, Riley RT, eds. *Managing Technological Change*. New York: Springer; 2004.
7. Campbell EM, Sittig DF, Ash JS, Guappone KP, Dykstra RH. Types of unintended consequences related to computerized provider order entry. *J Am Med Inform Assoc*. 2006;13(5): 547-556.
8. Gill RA, Walker JM. Optimizing inpatient care. In: Walker JM, Bieber EJ, Richards F, eds. *Implementing an Electronic Health Record System*. London: Springer; 2005.

9. Ash JS, Sittig DF, Campbell E, Guappone K, Dykstra RH. An unintended consequence of CPOE implementation: shifts in power, control, and autonomy. *AMIA Annu Symp Proc.* 2006:11-15.

10. Lorenzi NM, Riley RT. Critical design (redesign) issues. In: Lorenzi NM, Riley RT, eds. *Managing Technological Change: Organizational Aspects of Health Informatics.* New York: Springer; 2004.

11. Massaro TA. Introducing physician order entry at a major academic medical center: II. Impact on medical education. *Acad Med.* 1993;68(1):25-30.

12. Robbins SP, Judge T. *Organizational Behavior.* 12th ed. Upper Saddle River, NJ: Pearson/Prentice-Hall; 2007.

13. iHealthBeat, California HealthCare Foundation. *Online system reduces nurse documentation time.* http://www.ihealthbeat.org/index.cfm?Action=dspItem&itemID=98572; October 2002.

14. Wong DH, Gallegos Y, Weinger MB, Clack S, Slagle J, Anderson CT. Changes in intensive care unit nurse task activity after installation of a third-generation intensive care unit information system. *Crit Care Med.* 2003;31(10):2488-2494.

15. Case J, Mowry MM, Welebob E, First Consulting Group, California HealthCare Foundation. *The nursing shortage: can technology help?*, ihealth reports. Oakland, CA: California HealthCare Foundation; 2002.

16. Ammenwerth E, Mansmann U, Iller C, Eichstadter R. Factors affecting and affected by user acceptance of computer-based nursing documentation: results of a two-year study. *J Am Med Inform Assoc.* 2003;10(1):69-84.

17. Ammenwerth E, Eichstadter R, Haux R, Pohl U, Rebel S, Ziegler S. A randomized evaluation of a computer-based nursing documentation system. *Methods Inf Med.* 2001;40(2):61-68.

18. Liaskos J, Mantas J. Measuring the user acceptance of a web-based nursing documentation system. *Methods Inf Med.* 2006;45(1):116-120.

19. Banet GA, Jeffe DB, Williams JA, Asaro PV. Effects of implementing computerized practitioner order entry and nursing documentation on nursing workflow in an emergency department. *J Healthc Inf Manag.* 2006;20(2):45-54.

20. Poissant L, Pereira J, Tamblyn R, Kawasumi Y. The impact of electronic health records on time efficiency of physicians and nurses: a systematic review. *J Am Med Inform Assoc.* 2005;12(5):505-516.

21. Moody LE, Slocumb E, Berg B, Jackson D. Electronic health records documentation in nursing – nurses' perceptions, attitudes, and preferences. *Comput Inform Nurs.* 2004;22(6):337-344.

22. Kossman SP. Perceptions of impact of electronic health records on nurses' work. *Stud Health Technol Inform.* 2006;122:337-341.

23. Timmons S. The potential contribution of social science to information technology implementation in healthcare. *Comput Inform Nurs.* 2002;20(2):74-78.

24. Lorenzi NM, Riley RT. Managing change: an overview. *J Am Med Inform Assoc.* 2000;7(2):116-124.

25. Ash JS, Bates DW. Factors and forces affecting EHR system adoption: report of a 2004 ACMI discussion. *J Am Med Inform Assoc.* 2005;12(1):8-12.

26. Dykstra R. Computerized physician order entry and communication: reciprocal impacts. *Proc AMIA Symp.* 2002:230-234.

27. Österlund J, Lovén E. Information versus inertia: a model for product change with low inertia. *Syst Res Behav Sci.* 2005;22(6):547-560.

28. Ash JS, Stavri PZ, Kuperman GJ. A consensus statement on considerations for a successful CPOE implementation. *J Am Med Inform Assoc.* 2003;10(3):229-234.

29. Scott JT, Rundall TG, Vogt TM, Hsu J. Kaiser Permanente's experience of implementing an electronic medical record: a qualitative study. *BMJ.* 2005;331(7528):1313-1316.

30. Fischer D, Koziol R, Paust M, Soley J. *Aligning strategic project goals with organizational goals during technology implementations: hospitals and health systems.* CherryRoad Technologies, Inc. http://www.cherryroad.com/Documents/Whitepapers/Whitepaper_GoalAlignment.pdf; 2003.

31. Wood D. *Overcoming resistance to computerized EMR*. http://www.nursezone.com/include/PrintArticle.asp?articleid=13957&Profile=Hospital%20profiles; 2005.
32. Ammenwerth E, Kutscha U, Kutscha A, Mahler C, Eichstadter R, Haux R. Nursing process documentation systems in clinical routine – prerequisites and experiences. *Int J Med Inform*. 2001;64(2-3):187-200.
33. Bertelsen P, Madsen I, Hostrup P. Work flow analysis prior to implementation of an Electronic Patient Record (EPR): a method to disclose inconsistencies between the paper based medical record and the EPR. In: Fieschi M, ed. *Medinfo 2004: Proceedings of the 11th World Congress on Medical Informatics*. Fairfax, VA: IOS Press; 2004.
34. Koppel R, Metlay JP, Cohen A, et al. Role of computerized physician order entry systems in facilitating medication errors. *JAMA*. 2005;293(10):1197-1203.
35. Ahmad A, Teater P, Bentley TD, et al. Key attributes of a successful physician order entry system implementation in a multi-hospital environment. *J Am Med Inform Assoc*. 2002;9(1):16-24.
36. Young D. CPOE takes time, patience, money, and teamwork. *Am J Health Syst Pharm*. 2003;60(7):635, 639-640, 642 passim.
37. Parker P. Solutions success: clinical documentation technology. *Nurs Manage*. 2002;33(2):39-40.
38. InfoLogix Mobile Intelligence. *Computer wall mount workstation – Model 0-500 series*. http://www.healthcare.infologixsys.com/products/Products/Wall-Mount-Workstation/O-Computer-Wall-Mounts/Retractable-Wall-Desk-O-500/default.asp.

4
Implementation of an Electronic Prescription Writer in Ambulatory Care

Minhui Xie and Kevin B. Johnson

Oceanview Medical Center (OMC) successfully implemented a home grown, inpatient, computerized physician ordering entry system (CPOE). In early 2004, OMC launched a small pilot group as the need for a similar ordering entry system in ambulatory care was rising. Doctors, nurses, and programmers collaborated to develop an electronic prescription writer for ambulatory clinical setting. The system was named RxWriter and was designed to operate with the OMC electronic medical record system (OMCEMR, also home grown) to support prescription generation, easier communication of patient information, more efficient clinic workflow, automatic medication monitoring, and quality improvement.

Background

The OMC Environment

OMC is a tertiary care medical center located in Oceanview. As of 2007, OMC's clinical facilities include the 900-bed Oceanview Hospital (OH) and outpatient facilities in The Oceanview Clinic (TOC). TOC has more than 900 Medical Group physicians on staff, comprising over 95 outpatient specialty practices in several locations and provides a full range of diagnostic and treatment services. In 2007, OMC had over one million outpatient visits and 50,000 inpatient admissions.

OMC Strategic Plan Prioritized 'Patient Safety First'

The implementation of OMC projects was driven by the goals and the timeline defined in the OMC Strategic Plan. This strategic plan stated, "The first goal is that we want to be the best in class related to medication safety across the inpatient/outpatient continuum by the end of 2007."

RxWriter's Stakeholders and Team Organization

There are a variety of stakeholders involved in the electronic prescribing process. Each member plays a critical role in the complex process of prescription creation and management.[1]

L. Einbinder et al. (eds.), *Transforming Health Care Through Information: Case Studies*, Health Informatics, DOI 10.1007/978-1-4419-0269-6_4, © Springer Science+Business Media, LLC 2010

Stakeholders	Interests in electronic prescribing
Patient	Wants low cost, accurate, and safely written prescriptions meeting all possible constraints imposed by their insurance carrier (like on formulary or authorized if nonformulary)
Provider	Wants to create safe and therapeutically effective prescriptions, spending no more than 20 seconds for each prescription. Wants to write prescriptions that patients will take when dispensed.
Clerk	Wants to be sure that patient or pharmacy prescription requests are received and acted upon by prescriber or designee.
Nurse	Wants to be sure that patient or pharmacy prescription requests are received and acted upon by prescriber or designee. Also, if given a verbal order for a prescription (to give to pharmacy, etc.), the nurse wants that it is documented and "signed" by the issuing provider.
Pharmacists and associated staff in store-based and mail-order pharmacies	Want to be sure that prescription requests are received and acted upon by prescriber or designee. Want decision support (allergies, drug interactions, etc.) to ensure safe and effective medication administration. Want clear instructions on the prescription to ensure safe administration of what is dispensed.
Payer	Wants to create effective, safe, low cost, medically necessary prescriptions especially when insurer covers any of the prescription cost.
Researcher and management team in academic institutions, pharmaceutical and medical device manufacturers, and public health organizations	Want to make use of the data collected by electronic prescription writer, study clinical workflow related to prescribing process, optimize drug alert presentation, and achieve maximum patient safety.

The RxWriter development team includes one Project director, one Project manager, three Software developers, one Information Services Consultant (ISC), and one Quality Assurance (QA) Analyst. Their specific roles in the development of RxWriter are summarized as follows:

Team members	Specific roles
Project director	Leads the development efforts of the project, prioritizes application features on the basis of institutional initiatives, end user requests, and best practices (research, grants, etc.). Project director also drives the team to achieve consensus about the content and design of the solution among different project stakeholders.
Project manager	Works with the EMR team to communicate changes once the new features are ready for implementation. Project manager is also responsible for providing tutorials and organizing users' training.
Software developers	Work with all other team members and participate in the entire software lifecycle from design to implementation, configuration, and system maintenance.
The ISC	Is the liaison between the end users and the developers. He or she meets with the users to identify system requirements and translates those requirements into specifications the developers use to create the end product and various new features.
The QA analyst	Is responsible for making sure the RxWriter performs as intended. The QA analyst is intimately involved as the requirements evolve and begins testing the features very early in the development cycle. The QA analyst performs extensive tests once a version of RxWriter is ready to be disseminated to clinicians. The QA analyst also helps to prepare the new release for the users (engaging in change management practices).

The RxWriter team also includes a group of clinician consultants, in addition to other support staff who manage the system in which RxWriter is deployed. These staff include one Senior software developer from Information Technology Integration, one Project Manager from Incident management, one UNIX administrator, one WebLogic administrator, two database administrators, and specialists from HELP DESK support team and EMR support team.

RxWriter Implementation

The focus of this case study is the application development of RxWriter and the challenges it has been facing since being disseminated in an academic medical center with many other legacy systems already deployed.

RxWriter's Infrastructure and Dependencies

RxWriter was developed in house. It was created by the RxWriter development team using dynamic web pages based on the Java EE standards of Servlets and Java Server

Pages (JSP), and some Python for scripting. It's running in production using BEA Weblogic Java Application Server running on Sun Microsystems Solaris Servers.

Major Features and Accomplishments RxWriter Already Applied

RxWriter is a web-based outpatient prescription writer designed to create a safe and efficiently generated prescription. RxWriter contains a series of features designed to improve patient safety without compromising system speed or usability.

Complex prescribing features:RxWriter supports generic prescribing, formulary-based prescribing, and weight-based dosing (for pediatric patients). RxWriter provides therapeutic alternatives when, for example, a prescriber's preferred medication is not on the formulary for an insurer. It expands this approach by providing recommendations to the prescriber, after discussion with advanced user support team who identified the need. Besides producing prescriptions that are 100% legible, the application automatically looks for contraindications such as potential adverse reactions due to drug allergy or dosing mistakes. It supports pediatric dosing with weight-based prescribing guidelines, a built-in calculator, and dose-rounding heuristics to improve the dosing of liquid preparations. The application will issue an alert if anything appears wrong with a prescription.

Workflow Integration Features

RxWriter supports quick generation of prescriptions from current medication/medication favorites, quick refill/renewal process based on previous medications prescribed by user, local/remote Faxing/Printing and Pharmacy connection. RxWriter also is integrated with the OMC electronic health record system. It is designed to optimize clinicians' workflow. For instance, RxWriter may be used while reviewing a patient chart, writing an encounter summary, or sending a secure message. RxWriter prescriptions may be drafted by one provider, but completed by another. Communication is enhanced between the nurse and provider (or vice versa), the clinician and patient, and the clinician and pharmacy. Prescriptions created in RxWriter automatically show up in the patient's medication list and can be faxed to different pharmacies, improving communication throughout the Medical Center and between clinicians and pharmacists. In addition, notification emails can be generated and sent to the patient via the OMC patient portal, improving communication between clinicians and patients. RxWriter was recently challenged to respond to an incentive provided by a major insurer. In response to the inclusion of five new features, OMC received additional reimbursement. Those features were: weight-based dosing, generic based prescribing, formulary based prescribing, therapeutic alternatives, and dosing alerts.

RxWriter also provides support for research aimed at improving e-prescribing systems nationally; two grants have been obtained to explore ways to further enhance patient safety and mediation compliance on the basis of RxWriter. RxWriter creates an average of 50,000 prescriptions per month and is implemented in almost all outpatient clinical areas in OMC with over 900 users (including physicians, nurses, and pharmacists). In the future, RxWriter will provide other built-in decision support by checking each new prescription against a patient's other medications and known problems (diagnoses, laboratory results). The extended decision support will cover drug-drug interaction, drug-food interaction, drug-disease contraindication, drug-lab contraindication, drug-geriatric contraindication, drug-lactation contraindication, drug-pediatric contraindication, drug-side effect, duplicate ingredient/therapy, and other areas of decision support.

RxWriter adoption is an ongoing process.

Number of Prescriptions Generated	Number of Physicians (including attending and residents)
1–10	154
11–50	224
51–250	194
250+	44
Total	616

Prescriber Activity, January 2008

RxWriter Implementation Challenges

Some major issues have already arisen in the ongoing development of RxWriter. Not all users are enthusiastic about RxWriter's ultimate fate if substantial progress is not made to achieve the objectives defined in the Strategic Plan.

1. Adoption. RxWriter is implemented in almost all outpatient clinical areas in OMC. It has over 900 users and is averaging 2,500 prescriptions per day. Although the usage is increasing (it is estimated as 60,000 prescriptions per month by the end of 2008), the adoption of RxWriter is modest; the majority of clinicians are not using it for all their prescriptions. The RxWriter team is working hard to promote the usage of electronic prescribing in outpatient clinical areas including a clinic-rounding exercise launched in the early 2007. As there is no single institution-wide accepted ordering system in ambulatory care, we can only estimate the percentage of prescriptions created by RxWriter: OMC averages 4,500 outpatient visits per workday; if we assume that a patient receives two medications per visit on average, we postulate that about 30% prescriptions are created by RxWriter in the OMC outpatient clinics (2,500/9,000).
2. Adequate but clinical relevant decision support. RxWriter currently only provides drug-allergy and drug-dosing decision supports. Drug-drug interaction, drug-disease contraindication, drug-lab conflict, and other categories of alerts are excluded. The available allergy or dosing alert information is retrieved from a commercial drug knowledge database. There is no home-grown or fine-tuned drug knowledge database available for outpatient clinical setting.
3. The need to have other outpatient orderings systems. RxWriter only supports medication ordering. All other outpatient ordering, such as x-ray and pathology reports, has to be completed using other methods, which as of now continue to be paper-based.

It is not a trivial exercise to implement an electronic prescription writer system and adopt it in practice. Despite its promising benefits, adoption of such systems is still slow nationally. When adopted, usage rates in ambulatory care are low. Current estimates suggest that between 5 and 18% of clinicians are using electronic prescribing.[2,3] Although many potential difficulties should be considered in establishing an electronic prescription writer, such as leadership, financial cost, user interface design, training, and the resistance from clinicians (due to the fear of changes and negative impact to work flow), the authors of this study attempt to describe the challenges and barriers from two perspectives: technical challenges and political challenges

Technical Challenges

Historically, OMC hospitals have typically employed a "Best-of-Breed" healthcare IT implementation strategy, investing in the top IT products available for each specialty or department, which leads to communication and data integration issues. Major vendor or in-house systems continue to operate as components within OMC information architecture today, including the following:

- Patient demographic: home-grown Enterprise Patient Index (EPI) system
- Patient scheduling, registration and billing: commercial systems
- Clinic labs, Microbiology and Anatomic Pathology: commercial system
- Radiology: commercial system
- Cardiology: commercial system
- PACS (Picture Archiving and Communications System): commercial system
- Inpatient Ordering: homegrown InptOrder system
- Pharmacy Management: commercial system
- Electronic Patient Chart, physician documentation, message basket, reminder, consulting service: home-grown OMCEMR system
- Nursing Documentation: Commercial System

These systems vary by vendor, infrastructure, development platform, programming language, and database backend, but they provide general services that RxWriter relies on to generate a prescription, trigger a decision support alert, or to document a completed prescription. RxWriter's project director, manager, and developers have spent a large amount of time collaborating with different groups to reach the consensus, adopt the changes, and find the solutions for all rising issues.

Decision support functionality is one of the main reasons to adopt an electronic prescription writer; however, current knowledge bases often lead to inappropriate alerts that may be time consuming and even inaccurate in some cases. Because these alerts require intervention, they often have a negative effect on the adoption of e-prescribing and are therefore disabled. The turn-off of decision support modules inevitably hampers prescription writer's promise of reducing potential adverse drug events (ADE) and improving patient safety. Unfortunately, this is exactly what RxWriter experienced.

RxWriter currently only provides drug-allergy and drug-dosing decision supports. In one of the authors' feasibility experiments, a mock-up case with two diagnoses, two allergies, and ten medications can trigger 20 clinical drug alerts from a drug knowledge-base (Nov. 2003 version), provided that only two screening modules are used. A case with four diagnoses and 20 medications can trigger more than 150 clinical drug alerts, provided that 7 of 13 screening modules are used, and the time spent is 30+ seconds.

How to group, prioritize, and display these multiple drug alerts is another technical challenge to both application developers and clinicians.

Political Challenges

OMC is unique in its preference for in-house development and strong collaboration between clinicians and developers. OMC was ranked highest in a 2004 comparison of the strength and functionality of clinical enterprise information technology in use at 22 U.S. medical centers. Before the RxWriter project was initiated, OMC already had been implementing two well-known clinical applications: InptOrder and OMCEMR.[4–6] The success of these two applications and other in-house developed projects raised the standards/thresholds for RxWriter to achieve expected results. It also posed a heavy pressure on RxWriter development team.

The InptOrder is the clinical decision support and ordering interface for the inpatient services. Using protocols and guidelines (e.g., drug-lab test, drug-disease contraindication) developed and maintained by local clinical experts (who utilize the literature and national guidelines), InptOrder is highly effective in guarding patient safety, improving quality, and lowering costs associated with unwanted variability in health care.

The OMCEMR integrates patient data from multiple sources that include demographics, lab results, radiology/cardiology/pathology reports, physician notes, physician letters, discharge summaries, problem lists, medication log, patient indicators/alerts, inpatient/outpatient/ED census, and external test results. It provides access to the electronic patient clinical information from one screen; it allows various ways to record the patient's data; it supports related workflow via message basket, work list, new results, draft-and-sign, whiteboard, indicator, consulting service, etc. The OMCEMR brings patient-related information in detail, at the moment that the clinician treats the patient, record the data, and communicate other clinicians.

RxWriter is implemented using dynamic web pages based on Java technology. However, the electronic patient record system (EPR) that is integrated with RxWriter is designed and implemented using a totally different approach. This difference engenders substantial obstacles to data sharing between various parities. Consequently, seamless integration, new feature development, and change to reflect optimized clinic workflow were often delayed. Indisputably, from the date the RxWriter project was initialized, there existed diverging opinions about the project's architecture, goals, and priorities among different stakeholders, end-user groups, development teams, and members. It is quite normal to have diverging opinions in the institute but we know that the decisions made initially about the project's design had a large impact on the RxWriter project's success.

Options

In this case study, the authors described in-house efforts to develop an electronic prescription writer for outpatient setting and the challenges encountered during the development. Although RxWriter has been readily accepted by most of clinic units and more features are added every month, many physicians are still not using it frequently. The difficulties encountered during RxWriter development seem grounded in two main areas: technical issues and political issues. The technical limitations of the system led to the opinion that the application did not supply clinically relevant and adequate decision support in order to reduce medication errors, as it promised. The political challenges exacerbated these complications in such a way that system integration and maintenance were hampered. In fact, the steering committee has realized the obstacles and has decided to work over policy goals and detailed procedures before fulfilling patient safety for outpatient setting. Dynamically, the accomplishment of RxWriter objectives has been moved to late 2009 on the high-level road map.

So what are the options available for the development team to tackle development difficulties posed by technical and political challenges?

1. Upgrade RxWriter to an institute-wide accepted ambulatory ordering system. Such system will cover not only medications but also labs tests, radiology tests, cardiology tests, pathology tests, and treatments/therapies for outpatient clinics. RxWriter is one of the major components in achieving the institution's goal of medication safety. That is perhaps why the project was initially designed to order medications only in outpatient clinics because OMC already has InptOrder to enhance medication safety in inpatient setting. But RxWriter doesn't cover nonmedication orders, such as lab tests, radiology report, and treatment. For example, at the end of a patient visit, when tests are ordered and medications are prescribed, providers must use two systems (RxWriter and paper) which is both inconvenient and potentially less safe. One key to InptOrder and OMCEMR's success is that both applications are all-in-one like interfaces in inpatient ordering or patient chart areas. A clinician can order drugs, tests, and treatments from InptOrder for inpatient services. The success of InptOrder and OMCEMR is the best evidence for supporting an expanded role of RxWriter as an all-in-one ordering interface in outpatient clinics.

2. Take the value from InptOrder decision support rules. An electronic prescribing system that can provide relevant clinical alerts is essential for clinicians and hospital management to realize its value and voluntarily help to speed up the adoption. When the prescribing clinician is writing or editing a prescription, he/she wants the whole process to be quick, but he/she also wants to know if the prescription is appropriate for the clinical context. In OMC, clinical experts develop and maintain evidence-based knowledge bases including protocols and guidelines for ordering practice. InptOrder adopted this approach with good results and the application is applauded by clinicians. RxWriter could consider utilizing InptOrder decision support rules as RxWriter relies on a commercial drug knowledgebase that contains a large number of potentially irrelevant alerts. However, the InptOrder alert set is too constrained for the variety of medications that are prescribed to outpatients, thereby making it potentially unsafe, as prescribers may begin to rely on it, not realizing that it is not as inclusive as it should be. In response to this challenge, the RxWriter team has assembled a team of physicians, nurses, and pharmacists to review all the alerts in the knowledgebase and to filter out unnecessary ones. It is our hope that over time, the drug alerts will become more clinically relevant.

3. Adopt a platform/infrastructure similar to that of OMCEMR for better integration. InptOrder is programmed mainly using C/C++, OMCEMR is run on distributed servers, and programmed mainly using Perl. It seems that the success is unrelated to programming language and application architecture. But the authors of this study

disagree with such views. Prescription writer is not a segregated application, it needs to actively load and review patient archival data. These data are generated from multiple sources such as diagnosis, lab results, pathology reports, progress notes, and medication logs. They cover different service areas including inpatient, outpatient, and emergency departments, occupation health, and psychiatric hospital. OMCEMR is already an all-in-one interface for patient archival data from almost all sources. It is equally important that Prescription writer needs to fit workflow within clinical office. An electronic prescribing system that easily adapts to the workflow of all appropriate staff in the practice is critical to adoption. Once the prescribing clinician is writing or editing a prescription, various other tasks must be performed to complete the work. Workflow that needs to be considered includes printing, delivering, and communication with other clinicians/pharmacists. OMCEMR is developed to support various workflows by making the data available in all clinic locations and from a variety of sources. Hopefully, with increasing integration and system evaluation, RxWriter will leverage this approach and continue to succeed.

Questions

1. What were the problems that RxWriter program was intended to address? What will occur if RxWriter related goals defined in institutional strategic plan are not achieved?
2. If you are a strategic planner, what challenges do you envision for RxWriter?
3. What key factors contributed to RxWriter's successful development in OMC?
4. What key factors contributed to RxWriter's acceptance by clinicians in OMC?
5. Are there any potential issues you believe that the steering committee of RxWriter may not have initially considered?
6. If another outpatient group was planning to implement a similar electronic prescription writer, what are the most important experiences that they could learn from RxWriter of OMC?

Acknowledgments   We sincerely thank Dr. Nancy Lorenzi, Wendy Kiepek, Jeff Byrd, and Eric Boehme who provided data and suggestions during the course of development of this case study.

References

1. RxWriter development team. RxWriter Project High Level Design Document. 2006
2. Electronic Prescribing: *Toward Maximum Value and Rapid Adoption. Recommendations for Optimal Design and Implementation to Improve Care, Increase Efficiency and Reduce Costs in Ambulatory Care.* A Report of the Electronic Prescribing Initiative. eHealth Initiative. Washington, D.C. 2004.
3. Bell BS, Cretin S, Marken RS, Landman AB. A Conceptual Framework for Evaluating Outpatient Electronic Prescribing Systems Based on Their Functional Capabilities. *J Am Med Inform Assoc.* 2004;11(1):60–70.
4. Miller RA, Gardner RM, Johnson KB, Hripcsak G. Clinical decision support and electronic prescribing systems: a time for responsible thought and action. *J Am Med Inform Assoc.* 2005;12(4):403–409.

5. Miller RA, Waitman LR, Chen S, Rosenbloom ST. The anatomy of decision support during inpatient care provider order entry (CPOE): empirical observations from a decade of CPOE experience at Vanderbilt. *J Biomed Inform.* 2005;38(6):469–485.

6. Stead WW, Bates RA, Byrd J, Giuse D, Miller RA, Shultz EK. Case Study: The University Medical Center information management architecture. In: Van De Velde R, Degoulet P, eds. *Clinical Information Systems: A Component-Based Approach.* Springer, 2003.Section I. Managing change4. Implementation of an Electronic Prescription Writer in Ambulatory Care

5
Online Health Care: A Classic Clash of Technology, People, and Processes

JOHN BUTLER, DAN DALAN, BRIAN MCCOURT, JOHN NORRIS, and RANDALL STEWART

"I'm an old fashioned doc and I really fear and distrust where medicine is heading."

This statement, in an e-mail to all physicians at FutureCare Medical Group, epitomized the ambivalence many physicians had for On-Line Patient Services. "Me too," a partner chimed-in. "WE'LL GO BROKE!" e-mailed another. And so, a string of e-mails expressed frustration, doubt, and even shear refusal to participate in this major strategic initiative. Encouraging patients to send e-messages to unenthusiastic doctors would be a recipe for failure. Without physician support, the project would go nowhere. What was happening? What should be done?

Based on a real life scenario with some fictionalized details, the organization, individuals and email text presented in this paper have been altered to protect confidentiality.

Introduction

Cell phones, e-mail, and internet resources have changed traditional communication patterns, reducing the need for face-to-face communication. Simultaneously, more demanding work schedules and overbooked physician's appointments have increased the difficulty of making face-to-face, physician office visits. Therefore, online services offered by non-medical institutions (e.g., banks, airlines, and retail stores) have increased the public's expectations for services that should be made available online.[1]

As the workload for physicians continues to grow, uncompensated time for phone calls and e-mail exchanges is increasingly competing with compensated clinical time. Concurrently, diminishing payments for billable services have decreased the profit margins traditionally allocated for provision of uncompensated services such as phone calls or e-mail exchanges.

For patients to use telephone and e-mail services, providers lose clinical time and revenue. A possible solution for this zero-sum game is to bill for telephone calls and e-mail exchanges. This can be seen as a win-win situation for physicians (who are compensated for their time), for patients (who enjoy the convenience), and for third-party payers (who may pay less for an electronic visit than for an office visit). As such, the American Medical Association (AMA) has taken steps to change the culture toward billing for phone calls and electronic encounters.

L. Einbinder et al. (eds.), *Transforming Health Care Through Information: Case Studies*, Health Informatics, DOI 10.1007/978-1-4419-0269-6_5, © Springer Science+Business Media, LLC 2010

The AMA-developed provider guidelines for e-mail with patients,[2] established separate billing codes for telephone services, and in 2008 released a new code (99444) for billing for "online services."[3] The requirements for using the 99444 code do not distinguish between e-mail interactions or interactions via a web-based portal. This sets a low technological bar to bill for online services so that even small practices can potentially bill for e-mail interactions. Though the Center for Medicare and Medicaid Services (CMS) does not currently reimburse for this service some third-party payers have begun reimbursing online interactions.[4]

Our case study is FutureCare Medical Group, an 800 physician, fee-for-service primary care and multi-specialty group in a large metropolitan area. FutureCare utilizes an electronic health record that has been implemented over the last 5 years in 40 outpatient clinics. FutureCare leadership believes that on-line services will provide better and more efficient care, a more loyal patient population and allow the group to distinguish itself in the marketplace. This is in line with the stated mission, "To continually improve the health of its patients."

FutureCare culture encompasses a variety of issues that are important to understand when looking at changes that on-line service brings. Though this medical group is moderately supportive for innovation and prides itself as a leader in healthcare, most innovations remain centrally driven. Local risk is restricted and variation usually entails layers of discussion and approval. As in most healthcare groups, attention to detail is expected, especially for financial, service, and health outcomes, and particularly for publicly reported topics such as service levels, access, and specific healthcare measures. Leadership has recently recognized staff morale as a major issue and new initiatives are considered for their impact on work-life balance. Although team-based work is espoused, individuals are generally held accountable for their own clearly defined job roles. While the need for growth is recognized, particularly in profitable specialty areas and new service lines, staff attitudes mostly reflect need for a conservative approach in a mature, competitive marketplace with three other large medical groups in the metropolitan area.

Two years ago, after extensive discussions and work-flow redesign at a pilot clinic, an on-line health record interface was added, so that patients could review problem and medication lists, medical history, health maintenance, lab and imaging test results, access references, and send messages to their care team. For certain health concerns not requiring face-to-face encounter, patients can now initiate an "e-visit" as an alternative to a clinic visit. The retail cost established by the medical group for an e-visit is $35, but most patients would pay an office visit copay (for e-visits as defined by AMA). FutureCare reimburses physicians with 0.5 RVU for a billed e-visit.

E-visits make sense. Traditional clinic visits require patients to be away from home or work for an average of 3 hours; e-visits offer patients convenience and time savings. E-visits can be convenient for physicians as well. Asynchronous communication can be done at the physician's convenience, with no phone tag. Because the content of these messages is automatically entered in the electronic record, case documentation is more complete and requires no additional effort on the part of the provider.

However, physician surveys and focus groups indicated ambivalence toward on-line services. Some were worried about effects on the patient-physician relationship. While there were a number of early adopters, growth has been slow even though demographic studies indicate that about 80% of FutureCare patients use the Internet.

In order to increase patient participation a more determined effort was called for. The marketing department advised that a password and user name be presented by receptionists to all patients as they enter the clinic door as a "gift," a perk of being a FutureCare patient. Pinetree Clinic was asked to pilot the new process. Receptionists, nurses, physicians and even phlebotomists, were given scripts promoting the use of on-line services. Though some physicians and staff remained ambivalent, there was general agreement to proceed with this marketing strategy.

The Pinetree Clinic pilot failed. Only 21% of patients who had visited Pinetree Clinic were now registered, barely a measurable difference from the baseline of 20%. After 3 months of the pilot, the project was abandoned. What could be learned from this pilot effort? Project managers sought to understand physician sentiments.

Initiating and Evaluating Change

Shortly afterwards Dr. Proctor, Medical Director for FutureCare, sent out an email to the Primary Care Provider's group.

> From: G. Proctor, M.D., Medical Director, FutureCare Medical Group
>
> Sent: May 7, 2008 09:21:22 AM
>
> To: Primary Care Providers
>
> Subject: Advice needed-improving clinic efficiency
>
> We expect patients will start more e-visits now that the word is out. We are putting out a survey shortly asking you all how it's going.
>
> It seems there is no consistent way folks are handling e-mail and e-visits. So we are thinking a redesign around phone messages, e-mails, and e-visits. What do you all think? --G

Initiating and evaluating change are fundamental aspects of change management and include a variety of organizational behavioral issues.

Evaluating Change

It is important to communicate before a planned change, to solicit information as well as participation.[5] This simple e-mail fits well into the first step in Lewin's three step model (Unfreeze:Movement:Refreeze) for successful change.[5] The e-mail tells the members of the group that the status quo is being "unfrozen" by releasing the restraining forces and asking for input. Asking for an evaluation is a message that change is possible. Depending on the answers to the e-mail, driving forces may be identified as well.

However, evaluation of changes may also cause difficulties. Evaluation done very shortly after the last change will not allow sufficient time for the earlier changes to become "fixed." The change cycle may be drawn out, giving the opportunity for some employees to try to turn things back to the original process.[5]

Surveys are an important way to evaluate change. However, more structure[5] in this early message, may have elicited more constructive feedback and better addressed specific areas of concern. This message may have benefited by including more about what is going right with the project, appreciative inquiry,[5] and how the organization could use its strengths to make for better processes. The message would support team-work. The use of "we" when describing the implementers and "you all" for the survey recipients puts up barriers to team approaches.

Initiating Change

FutureCare is introducing a major conceptual change and with it the significant problems of process, role, technology, communication and other implications. This is huge change. This e-mail intends to begin a discussion about some general process issues, but as we will see, the responders end up talking about the deeper concepts as well.

The e-mail touches on Kotter's steps for implementing change,[6] introducing an urgent need for change and asking the recipients to help together to accomplish the vision of more patients using the service. It encourages people to come up with ideas to help it out. It is reassessing past changes; however, it does not really make a direct connection between the recent changes and success to the organization.

Part of Participative Leadership, as this e-mail displays, is asking your group advice on what to do.[7] However, e-mail may not be the best way to begin this conversation. The lack of time invested in writing an e-mail may be interpreted as that amount of caring. This message seems to be about a specific process, consistent workflow; as such it is displaying a transactional form of leadership. What may be needed is more empha-sis on transformational leadership.[7]

E-mail is not a rich channel for communication and does not provide a good support for emotional content.[7] The start of change can be a stressful time, face-to-face communication would be a better channel to handle the variety of issues

Individual Response to Change

Patient care organizations such as FutureCare are particularly complex and challeng-ing environments for new technologies or workflow methods to be adopted success-fully. The tension between running a business in a competitive market and provision of patient-centric care often appear at odds. Aligning the individuals with the diverse roles and backgrounds that make up a large organization and its patient population are a significant challenge. Understanding individual perspectives and responses to the change in the organization are critical to the successful implementation of e-visits. As the focus of this paper is the clinicians a key element from their perspective is that they find the daily interactions with patients' very rewarding.[8] Thus, when making a change to the patient care process that impacts this physician-patient interaction, even one aligned with the clinical mission of FutureCare, is difficult.

As we continue analysis of the individual behaviors revealed in the e-mail discus-sion, Dr. Banner has provided a particularly honest and self aware perspective...

From D. Banner, M.D. FutureCare Pinetree Clinic

Sent May 8, 2008 06:57:33 AM

To: Primary Care Providers

Subject: RE: Advice needed-improving clinic efficiency

I'm an old fashioned doc and I really fear and distrust where medicine is heading. Maybe we need to be on the front of all this electronic messaging, that it is good marketing, but I believe we shouldn't lose site of personal face-to-face meetings and the human touch. —B

Dr. Banner highlights a theme of growing disconnect between "medicine" and his personal medical practice. The fear, distrust and feeling of loss caused by changes to the medical establishment seem solely his burden. The conflict that arises from the organizational structure is obvious. The push towards an electronic medium for communication with patients is a widely understood business strategy with increasingly well defined return on investment and method to meet competition in the healthcare marketplace. Dr. Banner plays a role in the organization structure whose focus is on the service relationship with patients, and quality care is built on personal relationships that have heavy reliance on the human moment.[9] Even the best-designed electronic interactions do not match the communication possible between two people in physical presence.[10] This is in contrast to the ways other roles in the organization define success. Without effective opportunities for each department to be educated on the others' perspectives, an increase in distrust and resistance can be expected in the organization.

Resistance to change is natural. It must be appropriately taken into account when implementing any new system. Resistance is often overcome through education, opportunities for engagement in the change process, and negotiation among the roles in the group. For example, the business leadership has knowledge of details on the position of FutureCare in the market, competitor strategies, and other cost-benefit analysis of the proposed changes. The physicians have knowledge about interacting with patients, meeting their needs and quality medicine. From the physician's perspective, the use of an electronic intermediary with patients impinges on face-to-face communication. FutureCare needs to find a way to make the knowledge and value contributed by each of the roles visible to everyone. This education, ideally in participative forums, will allow individuals the opportunity to learn the perspectives and contributions of each group. These forums will also enable discussions (or negotiations) on the changes that shape implementation plans, thus it would include all stakeholders.

From: K.H. Dommer, M.D., FutureCare Medical Group

Sent: May 8, 2008 12:45:33 PM

To: Primary Care

Subject: RE: Advice needed-improving clinic efficiency

Yes, we need to spend time with patients, but some patients prefer e-visits.

BUT...I can't keep adding hours and I need to get PAID. We do enough free stuff around here as it is. Someone, patient? insurance? needs to pay for this stuff. Patients have already figured out how to avoid a co-pay by phoning in their questions. We need consistent guidelines on this or WE'LL GO BROKE! —KH

Negotiation becomes important when individuals recognize changes occurring. As the e-mail conversation continues, Dr. Dommer is ready to negotiate; he has recognized online physician services are going to be implemented and wonders how to make it sustainable The lack of payment is not only a business concern, it also inappropriately utilizes physicians. Without the education and participatory processes it would appear there was a lack of organizational value (and lower pay) placed on a physician's cognitive work.[11]

Attitudes can be characterized by using three interrelated components: cognitive, affective and behavioral.[12,13] The cognitive evaluation of the situation can be impacted by conveying the logical value of e-visits, such as the expected time efficiencies and earned revenue. A positive online experience that mimics positive personal interactions will support the affective feeling that the project is good. However, it is difficult to replicate a personal interaction with technology.[9,10] Lastly, behavioral components drive action. The actions of patients are the desired results of almost all clinical encounters. Enabling the right actions can increase adherence with e-visit policy, physician instructions and even beneficial health habits.

Motivation and Role Ambiguity

From: J. Myers, M.D., Pinewood Clinic

Sent: May 8, 2008 4:45:24 PM

To: Primary Care

Subject: RE: Advice needed-improving clinic efficiency

The market, and future, is with these electronic options, but I'm not going to give my pager number to my patients. We can't be expected to do this on our "off" hours. And 20 min of e-mail needs to pay as well as a 20 min office visit. Some doc's are having patients call so they can be billed.

Others are going back and forth with e-mail, some route to RN's, LPN's and Medical Office Assistants–how to handle these is as clear as mud. Oh, chronic care docs might get a lot of messages, but ED docs aren't — JM

Role conflict and ambiguous motivation is apparent in many of the preceding and following e-mail messages, the above message demonstrates these issues.

Myers relates role conflict in the form of "serving many masters." In the first sentence, Myers makes reference to "the market" and "the future" as reasons to use "electronic options" (e-visits). This impinges on the physicians' highly valued professional autonomy.[14-16] Myers continues with a reference to maintaining boundaries, an issue of growing importance to many physicians.[17]

Typical forces for change include competition, new technology, and cultural change. These are clear in the case for e-visits: competition for patients between FutureCare and other local providers, the developing technology allowing practical e-visits, and the public's cultural expectations for Internet-based services. These changes create goals.

The series of e-mail messages shows that the providers are unclear about the goals. Is the goal to increase revenue, save time, improve care, standardize processes, enhance efficiency, improve morale, or offer more convenient alternatives for patients?

While all of these goals are worthwhile, the ones measured are seen as the most important. The only quantifiable measure that the clinic is tracking is the proportion of patients using e-visits. In addition to being externally imposed, this goal has no practical significance to providers and is not directly sensible to them during the course of clinic visits.

Goal uncertainty hinders clear vision and increases the risk of role conflict. Unpredictability in medical practice makes the determination of the appropriate level of care (phone, e-mail, e-visit, face-to-face) inherently problematic.

Change Management

The e-mails continue with different, often opposing, contributions. Using the construct provided by Lewin's field theory[18] the e-mails can be viewed as positive or negative forces being exerted on the change being considered. Understanding the magnitude and directionality of views can help in the evaluation and handling of them as the changes move forward. The next exchange highlights a particularly vexing issue:

From: DB Coop, M.D. FutureCare Medical Group

Sent: May 8, 2008 4:45:24 P

To: Primary Care

Subject: RE: Advice needed-improving clinic efficiency

The EMR and on-line services is all about having good access to information. Why can't I quickly get access to our outside allergist's notes and how about them accessing us? I know they may lack our tools, but we should be more integrated.—DB

Change management is a structured approach to transitioning individuals, teams, and organizations from a current state to a desired future state,[19] but what if that desired state is in flux? What of the third party clinic doctors that thrive on consultant work for FutureCare patient care? They may be willing but lack computer technology resources. The opposing view exemplified above may not impact the advancement (or retreat) of the change but does effect the scope. It also serves to increase the conflict and stress associated with being in the "unfrozen" state of change.

The FutureCare online project is a planned change, and the chief forces for change involve competition and technology.[20] Uncertainty exists for some clinic providers, but overall, they have the awareness, desire, knowledge, and ability to change. They are leveraged by financial gains and prestige through possession of leading edge technology within a highly competitive market. Buy-in for online services will be easily sustained and reinforced; if patients use the services and third party payers reimburse physician efforts. Cost and complexity of technology appear to be the major hurdles. However, this may not be true of physicians outside FutureCare that may not have EMR,[21] or they lack compatible systems needed to provide the online services on the FutureCare EMR platform.

To achieve online implementation, the primary challenge is to adhere to classic project constraints of scope, quality, and time and budget characteristic of project management.[19,22] Dr. Coop's e-mail hijacks the e-mail thread and lets everyone know that they will need to have further negotiation and compromise. Ideally they can create a win-win situation so that consulting physician buy-in is achieved.

From: Dan D., M.D. Allergy & Asthma consultant to FutureCare

Sent: May 12, 2008 8:00 AM

To: FutureCare management

Subject: FutureCare online participation

Other health systems in similar situations have leveraged technology advances and relaxation of the Stark laws[23] to create greater efficiencies and satisfaction in their online services. FutureCare online service is not just e-mail; it falls within the definition of a personal health record.[24] There is a continuum between an EHR and a PHR[25,26] such as the recent offering by Kaiser Permanente Health Connect,[27] who reported early and high enrollment from patients and physicians, high satisfaction and opportunities to save time and increase co-payments. FutureCare's specialists are a key to increasing quality care in our community and it doesn't do either of our businesses good to be isolated. Let's discuss further. —Dan

While Dan's e-mail does not report all the technology options and growing evidence that support adopting the requirements of consulting physicians it does move the project forward with a shift toward integrative bargaining.[28] This approach will more likely result in both parties being satisfied with project's scope and outcome. The next e-mail adds another, but similarly restraining, perspective.

From: G. Clarke, Analyst III FutureCare IT

Sent: May 8, 2008 6:47:01 PM

To: Primary Care

Subject: RE: Advice needed – improving clinic efficiency

OK, we went over this already and have all e-mail and e-visits going to Office Assistants to start, then RN's.

Our intent was to grease the way for the provider so they could review information gathered by triage. Some RN's, though, thought we may have been delaying care waiting for patients to convert e-mails to e-visits. Some of the docs didn't want to charge for the e-visits. —GC

Clarke gives a succinct answer to the main technical process under question. Clarke's e-mail is quite different from the rest. Why is it so different? Is it a helpful addition to the thread?

Clarke is from the IT department. IT staff are used to quicker results,[16] are more concerned with the information system performance, and are not as aware of the clinician's culture. Clarke's well meaning message, may not be interpreted by clinicians as such. The simple "we went through this already" denotes impatience with the clinicians. Clarke only talks about process and does not address the emotions behind people's concerns nor mention the other issues they have been posting. The terse wording shows a lack of empathy. Such a message may elicit mistrust. If this is the case, the implementation will be in trouble.[29,30] The message conveys a sense of dependency for both I.T. and clinicians. Dependency creates power relationships[31] and possible areas for more conflict.

Management and Leadership

From: G. Procter, M.D., Medical Director FutureCare Medical Group

Sent: May 9, 2008 6:55:47 AM

To: Primary Care

Subject: RE: Advice needed – improving clinic efficiency

Overall thoughts- we need to work together to make the system work for us and our patients.

We need to make sure messages are done efficiently, with the right person doing the right work, that they get paid for the time they work...consistency is also key...but we have leading clinics that help point the way. Birchwood clinic has defined work flows well and is registering many new on-line patients with enthusiastic staff.

Our patients are busy and there are alternatives to us (outside urgent care clinic with great access are competing!) so we need to pursue this. I don't think we will be flooded with messages, but we should build the ark now!

Talk to your primary care champions, they are working with the manager of online services to include things like templates, and a new webpage that spells out for patients the difference between an e-visit and an e-mail. — GP

Dr. Proctor once more enters in on the discussion. Dr. Proctor's quick summary shows understanding of the responses and reiterates why all this is important. The e-mail also gives everyone the appropriate persons to as well as identifies some small, but possibly significant changes coming. Dr. Proctor also mentions a success...

In contrast to the Pinetree pilot, the Birchwood Clinic made steady progress in registrations. Active on-line patients rose to 37%, with some care teams approaching 50% of their patients using on-line services. This happened with seemingly little authoritarian leadership. Physicians found efficiency in working e-visits into their day, and releasing lab tests on-line. Clinic leadership encouraged all staff to sign up and use the online services. One of the receptionists was thrilled by the on-line services. "Why would not patients want to use this?" she said. She talked enthusiastically with patients as they checked in for appointments. Receptionists were worried about losing their jobs, so they were inspired to hear a vision where they would have more involvement with healthcare delivery.

Medical organizations are complex adaptive systems (CAS).[32,33] The word "complex" refers to the many connections and relationships between agents of a system. With its independent thinking workforce, performing many tasks for patients with widely varying needs, a healthcare organization is certainly complex. Healthcare outcomes are dependent on far more than the aggregate of isolated individual performances. Health informatics, internet based information sources, and now on-line communication with informed patients have dramatically changed and intensified these interactions.

Stacey[25] describes a decision matrix for analyzing policy making in such systems. This analysis would predict that in issues for which there is universal agreement and the direction is clear, management by rules and standardized processes would suffice. However, issues for which agreement is not universal, and the direction is still developing (such as the use and role of on-line services) call for CAS management principles.

In complex adaptive systems a "good enough" vision is effective. Acceptable boundaries are made clear. Emergent processes will appear.[34,35] Individuals, their experiences and relationships create the chemistry for change. At the Birchwood Clinic, a few individuals (physicians for whom on-line services worked) provided catalyst. Small management interventions can lead to large changes. This so called "butterfly effect" is the notion that a butterfly moving its wings in Brazil could create subtle air currents that could, through a chain of events, eventually spawn a tornado in Texas.[36,37] In the case of Birchwood Clinic, simply encouraging some staff to use on-line services as consumers, contributed to growing enthusiasm for this health care tool.

Strategic Planning for FutureCare

A series of e-mails between physicians alerts us to a range of physician concerns. Every e-mail expresses a different concern. Some are concerned with patient convenience, and others are concerned about improving care, increasing revenue, standardizing processes, using time efficiently, or discrepancies between business and healthcare goals. The vision for how e-visits will contribute to achieving the corporate mission is at best ambiguous. The vision in this case must articulate FutureCare as a leading-edge organization willing to incorporate the newest technology to improve the health of its patients and community. Goals must satisfy the worries that skeptical physicians and other staff have about quality of care, physician-patient relationship, time boundaries, and fair reimbursement.

Kotter's steps for implementing change provide a useful framework for planning.[6] Communication to physicians must make a case for urgent need to change. Influential physicians must take the lead. Physician opinion leaders along with other stake-holders (including patients) must be involved in decision making and planning. Business goals are important but a case must be made by and for clinicians that health care will be benefited. Physician efficiency must be supported through adequate resources. Physician reimbursement must be fair.

A "good enough vision" that includes the perspective of many stakeholders, must be articulated throughout. Local innovation should be supported and barriers broken down. The technology is rapidly changing, and strategy must include flexible, nimble processes that stakeholders are involved in developing, and provisions for whatever the future may hold. Short term wins that move in the direction of new vision will provide momentum. Consolidate improvements, and reinforce changes by pointing out how change leads to success. Our rapidly changing healthcare environment is fraught with uncertainty. It is a leader's great challenge to create a vision that aligns organizational forces, while making the environment fertile for innovation and adaptation. As Gareth Morgan observed, "Farmers don't grow crops, they create the conditions in which crops grow."[32]

The organization, individuals, and email text presented in this paper have been altered to protect confidentiality in this real-life scenario.

References

1. Melzer SM, Poole SR. Reimbursement for telephone care. *Pediatrics*. 2002;109(2):290-293.
2. Chin T. AMA delegates sort through patient e-mail issues. At: http://www.ama-assn.org/amednews/2000/07/10/tesb0710.htm. Accessed 12.05.08.
3. American Medical Association. *Current Procedural Terminology CPT 2008 Standard Edition*. Chicago: AMA; 2007.
4. Porter S. New, revised CPT codes target online, telephone services. At: http://www.aafp.org/online/en/home/publications/news/news-now/practice-management/20080229cptcodes.html. Accessed 12.05.08.
5. Robbins SP, Judge TA. *Organizational Behavior*. 12th ed. Upper Saddle River, New Jersey: Pearson Prentice Hall; 2007:640-658.
6. Kotter JP. *Leading Change*. Boston: Harvard Business School Press; 1996.
7. Robbins SP, Judge TA. *Organizational Behavior*. 12th ed. Upper Saddle River, New Jersey: Pearson Prentice Hall; 2007:378-416.
8. Gunderson L. Physician burnout. *Ann Intern Med*. 2001;135(2):145-148.
9. Hallowell EM. The human moment at work. *Harv Bus Rev*. 1999;77(suppl 1):58-64, 66.
10. Deladisma AM, Cohen M, Stevens A, et al. Do medical students respond empathetically to a virtual patient? *Am J Surg*. 2007;193(6):756-760.
11. Poses R. More on physician reimbursement, CMS, the AMA's RVS Update Committee (RUC) The healthcare blog. At: http://www.thehealthcareblog.com/the_health_care_blog/2008/05/more-on-physici.html. Accessed 12.05.08.
12. Robbins SP, Judge TA. *Organizational Behavior*. 12th ed. Upper Saddle River, New Jersey: Pearson Prentice Hall; 2007:75.
13. Breckler SJ. Empirical validation of affect, behavior, and cognition as distinct components of attitude. *J Pers Soc Psychol*. 1984;47(6):1191-1205.
14. Ash J, Sittig DF, Campbell E, Guappone K, Dykstra R. An unintended consequence of CPOE implementation: shifts in power, control, and autonomy. *AMIA Annu Symp Proc*. 2006;11-15.
15. Landon B. Changes in career satisfaction among primary care and specialist physicians, 1997–2001. *J Am Med Inform Assoc*. 2003;289:442-449.
16. Reinertsen JL. Zen and the art of physician autonomy maintenance. *Ann Intern med*. 2003; 138:992-995.
17. Williams ES, Konrad TR, Linzer M, et al. Refining the measurement of physician job satisfaction: results from the Physician Worklife Survey. *Med Care*. 1999;37(11):1140-1154.
18. Lorenzi NM, Riley RT. *Managing Technological Change: Organizational Aspects of Health Informatics*. 2nd ed. New York: Springer; 2004:140-141.
19. Wikimedia Foundation. Change management (people). At: http://en.wikipedia.org/wiki/Change_management_%28people%29. Accessed 13.06.08.

20. Robbins SP, Judge TA. *Organizational Behavior*. 12th ed. Upper Saddle River, New Jersey: Pearson Prentice Hall; 2007:645-646.
21. Ackerman K. Report finds low EHR adoption rates. iHealthBeat. Oct. 16, 2006. At: http://www.ihealthbeat.org/articles/2006/10/12/Report-Finds-Low-EHR-Adoption-Rates.aspx?a=1 Accessed 13.06.08.
22. Wikimedia Foundation. Project management. At: http://en.wikipedia.org/wiki/Project_management June 13, 2008
23. Center for Medicaid & Medicate Services. At: http://www.cms.hhs.gov/physicianselfreferral/downloads/cms-ao-2008-01.pdf Accessed 13.06.08.
24. Markle Foundation. A common framework for personal health information. At: http://www.connectingforhealth.org/commonframework/docs/P9_NetworkedPHRs.pdf June 13, 2008.
25. Evans C, Marshall P, Derman J, Zeiger R. Platforms and personal health applications: what is the tipping point for interoperability? Panel presentation at: AMIA 2008 Spring Conference; 2008 May 29-31; Phoenix.
26. Jones T, Reti SR, Jenkins M, Bates DW, Zuckerman AE. Addressing the challenges of using PHR in the primary care setting, Panel presentation at: AMIA 2008 Spring Conference; 2008 May 29-31; Phoenix.
27. Kaiser Permanente. Kaiser permanente EHR system facts-KP HealthConnect electronic health record. At: http://www.kphealthconnectq4update.org. Accessed 13.06.08.
28. Robbins SP, Judge TA. *Organizational Behavior*. 12th ed. Upper Saddle River, New Jersey: Pearson Prentice Hall; 2007:517.
29. Ash JS, Stavri PZ, Kuperman GJ. A consensus statement on considerations for a successful CPOE implementation. *J Am Med Inform Assoc*. 2003;10(3):229-234.
30. Lapointe L, Rivard S. Getting physicians to accept new information technology: insights from case studies. *CMAJ*. 2006;174(11):1573-1578.
31. Robbins SP, Judge TA. *Organizational Behavior*. 12th ed. Upper Saddle River, New Jersey: Pearson Prentice Hall; 2007:474.
32. Zimmerman B. *Edgeware. Insights from Complexity Science for Health Care Leaders*. Irving, Texas: VHA Publishers; 1998.
33. Plsek P, Greenhalgh T. The challenge of complexity in health care. *BMJ*. 2001;323:625-628.
34. McDaniel RR, Jordan ME, Fleeman BF. Surprise, surprise, surprise! A complexity science view of the unexpected. *Health Care Manage Rev*. 2003;23(3):266-278.
35. Miller WI, McDaniel RR, Crabtree BF, Stange KC. Practice jazz: understanding variation in family practices using complexity science. *J Fam Prac*. 2001;50(10):872-878.
36. Stacy R. The science of complexity: an alternative perspective for strategic change processes. *Strategic Management Journal*. 1995;16(6):477-495.
37. Lorenz E. *The Essence of Chaos*. Seattle WA: University of Washington Press; 1993. Section I. Managing Change5. Online Health Care: A Classic Clash of Technology, People, and Processes

Section II
Patient Safety

Patient Safety 71
  Joan S. Ash

Chapter 6
A Dungeon of Dangerous Practices 73
  Andrew Amata, Allen Flynn, Michelle Morgan, Teresa Smith,
  and Mary Tengdin

Chapter 7
Different Sides of the Story 83
  Allison B. McCoy

Chapter 8
Barcode Medication Administration Implementation
  in the FIAT Health system 85
  Linda Chan, William Greeley, Don Klingen, Brian Machado,
  Michael Padula, John Sum, and Angela Vacca

Chapter 9
H.I.T. or Miss 97
  James McCormack, Bimal R. Desai, Jennifer Garvin,
  Randal Hamric, Kirk Lalwani, Andi Lushaj,
  Alexey Panchenko, Deborah Quitmeyer, and JoAnna M. Vanderhoef

Patient Safety

JOAN S. ASH

Health information technology (HIT) has been promoted as an effective mechanism for instilling safety into the health care system. A series of Institute of Medicine reports has dramatically called attention to safety issues in American hospitals, and suggested strategies, many of which include HIT, for addressing these issues.[1-4] There is indeed evidence that HIT can help the situation, especially for medication management. From the decision about what medication to order to the administration of that medication, the process from beginning to end can be assisted by electronic systems. Most medication errors occur at either the physician ordering stage (39%) or the nurse administration stage (38%).[5] Computerized provider order entry (CPOE) can improve legibility, and provide an opportunity for the clinician to receive help through clinical decision support systems, thereby helping to reduce errors at this early stage. Checks can be built into the system so that the system will identify a danger, such as an order for a drug to which the patient is allergic, and let the provider, or another responsible person such as a pharmacist, know. At the end of the entire medication process, the actual administration of the medication might be monitored through a bar code medication administration (BCMA) system, thus reducing errors at this final stage. Using such a system, the nurse scans a bar code on a bracelet on that patient's wrist, and a bar code on the drug's packaging. This provides a final opportunity for information about the particular patient to be checked against information about the drug so that the nurse can be alerted about a possible problem. Like a grocery check out system at the market, the magic of such technology can make our lives easier, but unlike the supermarket system, it can also cause physical harm if the system fails.

Reason has outlined the memorable Swiss cheese model of safety, which draws an analogy between holes in slices of Swiss cheese that normally would not all line up, but which would line up once in a while when circumstances were right. Without any blocks or checks and balances, an error could make it all the way through the system and harm a patient.[6] Fortunately, in medicine, especially in the inpatient environment, there are many checks and double checks. A hospital that has both CPOE and BCMA could expect to block most potential medication errors, although some medication administration discrepancies will likely persist unless additional measures are taken.[7] Neither CPOE nor BCMA is foolproof, and both suffer from both unintended consequences[8,9] and workarounds.[10]

The four cases presented here emanate from four different organizational settings, but they have a good deal in common. All of the organizations are working hard to improve patient safety by implementing informatics solutions for avoiding errors in the medications process. One case has as its focus the dilemma about over-alerting in a CPOE system. While alerts can be effective in preventing misguided orders, they can also cause "alert fatigue" or the "crying wolf" syndrome in which a clinician ignores a useful alert, not noticing it among those he considers useless and annoying. Two cases concern plans for implementing BCMA in response to "sentinel events," individual incidents that caused harm to patients. Like CPOE implementation, BCMA is a large organizational change impacting many areas of the hospital. These cases uncover the complexities, and offer some strategies for identifying and addressing the issues. Finally, the HIT or Miss case offers a picture of the future when hospitals will have multiple systems to safeguard the medication process. In this case, a string of unintended consequences related to system downtime leads to information system-induced harm, which has been referred to as e-Iatrogenesis.[11]

References

1. Kohn LT, Corrigan JM, Donaldson MS. *Eo Err is Human: Building a Safer Health System.* Washington, DC: National City Press; 2000.
2. Hurtado M, Swift E, Corrigan JM. *Envisoning the National Health Care Quality Report.* Washington, DC: National Academies Press; 2001.
3. Crossing the Quality Chasm: A New Health System for the 21st Century. Washington, DC: National Academies Press; 2002.
4. Aspden P, Corrigan JM, Wolcott J, Erickson SM. *Patient Safety: Achieving a New Standard for Care.* Washington, DC: National Academies Press; 2004.
5. Leape L, Bates DW, Cullen DJ, et al. Systems analysis of adverse drug events. *JAMA.* 1995;274:35-43.
6. Reason JT. *Human Error.* Cambridge, MA: Cambridge University Press; 1990.
7. FitzHenry F, Peterson JF, Arrieta M, Waitman LR, Schildcrout JS, Miller RA. Medication dministration discrepancies persist despite electronic ordering. *J Am Med Inform Assoc.* 2007;14(6):756-764.
8. Ash JS, Sittig DF, Poon EG, Guappone K, Campbell E, Dykstra RH. The extent and importance of unintended consequences related to computerized physician order entry. *J Am Med Inform Assoc.* 2007;14:415-423.
9. Patterson ES, Cook RI, Render ML. Improving patient safety by identifying side effects from introducing bar coding in medication administration. *J Am Med Inform Assoc.* 2002;9(5):540-553.
10. Koppel R, Wetterneck T, Telles JL, Karsh BT. Workarounds to barcode medication administration systems: their occurrences, causes, and threats to patient safety. *J Am Med Inform Assoc.* 2008;15(4):408-423.
11. Weiner JP, Kfuri T, Chan K, Flwles JB. E-Iatrogenesis: the most critical unintended consequence of CPOE and other IT. *J Am Med Inform Assoc.* 2007;14(3):387-388; discussion 389.Section II.   Patient SafetySection II.   Patient Safety

6
A Dungeon of Dangerous Practices

Andrew Amata, Allen Flynn, Michelle Morgan,
Teresa Smith, and Mary Tengdin

American hospitals are sometimes unsafe. This is not news to the staff at Santiago Health. In fact, the leadership at Santiago Health, a three-hospital system with one large hospital campus and two smaller satellite hospitals, is keenly aware of the indictments of the quality of current medical practices published by the Institute of Medicine. When it comes to medication use, Santiago Health's leaders know they have to solve many safety and billing problems. The organization attempts to mobilize its staff to create a multidisciplinary team to address medication safety. The system's organizational value of achieving excellence bolsters this work.

Santiago Health's main campus is the Santiago Care Centers (SCC). The SCC includes a 556-bed hospital, a cancer center, a cardiac care center, and an outpatient surgery center. Dr Trubelli, a compassionate pediatrician and a former Chief of Staff of the SCC, is now the Medical Director of Information Systems (IS) for Santiago Health. He has witnessed and been forced to explain too many medical errors during his career. He desperately wants to implement a system to bar code medications in advance of administration. Such systems provide nurses with electronic verification of all drug orders at the bedside. Scanning medication bar codes effectively prevents medication errors.

The SCC Pharmacy department also wants to provide patients with the extra measure of safety offered by using bar codes on medications. The struggle for Pharmacy is that no clear strategy exists for bar coding every medication. The unknown dimensions of the problem have created anxiety within the Pharmacy management team. In order to successfully bar code all doses, several new packaging, compounding, and delivery technologies will compete for simultaneous resources during implementation. Dramatic changes to pharmacy technician workflow must accompany these new systems. Pharmacy billing changes will result from dose charging at administration. Furthermore, the Pharmacy department has difficulty sharing its technical needs with Santiago Health's IS staff. One problem is that Pharmacy does not understand the varying roles and responsibilities within the IS department.

Nursing will also undergo some changes. Santiago Health has yet to formally approach the nursing staff with the bar coding idea. Some nurses and nurse administrators may be aware of the proposal. However, it is clear that staff nurses do not fully understand the major changes in nursing practice required to use bar coding at the point of care.

The issues here are more organizational than technical. Unspoken conflicts seem to exist between Pharmacy and Nursing, between Santiago Health leaders and lower level managers, and between IS personnel and Pharmacy. The Pharmacy department may be

L. Einbinder et al. (eds.), *Transforming Health Care Through Information:*
Case Studies, Health Informatics, DOI 10.1007/978-1-4419-0269-6_6,
© Springer Science+Business Media, LLC 2010

the site of internecine conflicts among its coordinators, pharmacists, and pharmacy technicians. The Nursing staff members may resist the bar coding initiative if they believe that this new system will overwhelm their workflow and disrupt the care they provide.

Background: A Harmful Event

Recently, Mrs. Robbin G. Smith, a 56-year-old dialysis patient, presented to the SCC emergency room with fever, chills, and signs of infection. Caregivers decided to treat Mrs. Smith with several antibiotics including low doses of Gentamicin. High blood levels of Gentamicin can damage one's hearing. Therefore, it was essential to draw routine blood samples to monitor Mrs. Smith's Gentamicin therapy. Staff explained precautions to Mrs. Robbin G. Smith and her husband, Jim Smith, a safety engineer for a Fortune 500 shipping company. After several hours in the Emergency Department, SCC staff admitted Robbin G. Smith to the hospital, room 5020.

When Mrs. Robbin G. Smith arrived on the fifth floor from the emergency room, another patient with a very similar name, Robin C. Smith, was undergoing treatment in room 5012 for pneumonia. Robin C. Smith, a 48-year old with no chronic health issues, was receiving large doses of intravenous Gentamicin once a day.

Several e-mails circulated on the fifth floor and in the Pharmacy department to alert hospital staff that both Robbin G. Smith and Robin C. Smith were inpatients at the SCC. The purpose of the communication was to prevent medical errors.

One evening, at 6:00 p.m., a Santiago nurse was preparing medications when she noticed an IV for Robbin G. Smith lying on the floor of the medication room. She called the Pharmacy and asked them to send a replacement dose of "Mrs. Smith's Gentamicin."

The Pharmacy technician who took the nurse's call did not notice there were two different Smiths on the fifth floor. The technician printed a label for a large replacement dose of Gentamicin for Robin C. Smith. Disastrously, a misalignment of Pharmacy's label printer cut off the last two digits of the room number on the right side of the label.

In order to make up for a perceived Pharmacy delivery mistake, the replacement Gentamicin arrived on the fifth floor, STAT, by pneumatic tube. Although the nurse administering the IV looked at the label, Robbin G. Smith received Robin C. Smith's entire daily dose of Gentamicin in error.

Twelve hours later, lab results indicated toxic levels of Gentamicin in Mrs. Robbin G. Smith's blood. At that point, the mistake became apparent. Unfortunately, as a result of this mishap, Mrs. Robbin G. Smith suffered very significant hearing loss. During the discussions of the incident with the Smith family, Mr. Kevin Dininger, pharmacist and Pharmacy operations manager, noted the anger and frustration on Jim Smith's face and the terrible sadness expressed by his wife. Kevin Dininger will never forget the comment Jim Smith made in complete exasperation, "This is not a hospital! It's a dungeon of dangerous practices!"

Organizational Overview

In the Santiago Health Organization, the two primary groups affected by the bar coding initiative are Physician Services, which includes the Information Services department and the implementation team, and Patient Care Services, which includes Nursing and Pharmacy. Leaders of both groups report directly to the president and CEO of Santiago Health. Others reporting to the president and CEO include Risk Management, the COO, and Administrative Services.

The primary physician advocate for the bar coding at the point of care (BPOC) initiative is Dr Trubelli. He is a vocal champion of this new technology. He believes it will substantially reduce the medical errors that harm his organization and its patients. His authority includes groups that are responsible for the scheduling, design, and roll-out of the BPOC system. Dr Trubelli sees no significant roadblocks to the implementation of BPOC. When asked recently about any tensions between groups or departments, he replied, "The majority of staff I have worked with amongst all disciplines are all very supportive of bar coding. I don't believe we will meet with much resistance." Dr Trubelli has worked at Santiago for 23 years.

An important role in the implementation of any new technology is the IS Director, a position held by Jen Goodman. Jen reports directly to Dr Trubelli. Jen is excited about the promise of bar coding but is understandably concerned about the details of the implementation. Her particular concerns focus on hardware logistics and system usability. Jen is easy to approach. Moreover, she has earned respect from Dr Trubelli and those reporting to her. She is an army Reservist Major and a graduate of Massachusetts Institute of Technology. She participated in the implementation of an army BPOC system one year ago. The structure at Santiago is slightly different from the army hierarchy she became accustomed to during her military service.

In Jen Goodman's group are both the BPOC implementation team and the Desktop and Device Services group managed by Carl Desco. The implementation team is made up of four individuals who handle the project management, support, and training for BPOC. The BPOC initiative competes with other IS projects. Therefore, 0.5 FTE is the most the implementation team could allocate to the BPOC project.

Carl Desco manages the Desktop and Device Services group, comprised of non clinical, technical employees who deploy and support hardware, devices, and a wireless network throughout the organization. Carl's focus is on providing excellent service and 100% network availability. Carl views the BPOC as something new for his group to support. However, Carl thinks the BPOC initiative is no different from any other new device requirement. He is not involved in software usability issues because he knows the implementation team has ownership of this area. He would like to see that the project schedule includes time and resources for a beta test period before the BPOC system goes into full production.

Carl Desco is also married to one of the individuals in his group. They have been working together at Santiago for seven years. Carl tries not to show favoritism to his wife, but they sometimes leave the other members of Desktop services out of the loop.

Two other clinically oriented groups affected by BPOC are Nursing and Pharmacy. Both of these groups, along with Nutrition, Radiology, and Laboratory Services, are part of the Patient Care Services division. It is important to note the number of organizational levels that separate a unit nurse from a staff pharmacist. Unit nurses are the most frequent users of any BPOC system and staff pharmacists will be the first called when problems arise. The Pharmacy Operations Manager, Kevin Dininger, is worried that stakeholder voices will go unheard during the design and implementation of BPOC. He believes that rapid implementation is unwise. Kevin is aware of the current limitations of bar coding, including the workflow impact to his staff. For example, pharmacists will be required to manually bar code the majority of commercially available medications. Not surprisingly, his staff is well versed in the issues and echoes his sentiments. Kevin Dininger has little contact with Jen Goodman. He has not had the opportunity to share his concerns about the timeline of the BPOC system rollout. Kevin has heard that Jen participated in an army hospital rollout for bar coding, and, therefore, he has decided to schedule a brief meeting with Jen to talk about the Pharmacy issues he anticipates in order to implement BPOC at Santiago Health.

Some of the SCC nurses have heard about the bar coding project and have expressed interest, curiosity, and fear. To date, many staff nurses are unaware of the changes that are looming. Others do not feel empowered to make their opinions known. Fortunately, the coordinators in Pharmacy, Cindy Marshall, RN and Andrew Foor, RPh are considering nursing issues and discussing the likely impact of BPOC on the staff nurse. One reason for this is that the Pharmacy and Nursing departments have a history of working collaboratively. Andrew Foor, the Pharmacy Informatics Coordinator, is clearly concerned that the Pharmacy group maintains credibility with Nursing. He remembers a recent, botched software upgrade by Pharmacy that caused problems for the nurses. Thankfully, the trust between these two groups did not suffer irrevocable damage. Nurses continue to report that the Pharmacy Department listens well and responds to their feedback. Cindy Marshall was once a Nurse Educator for the Intensive Care Unit and she still keeps in touch with her Nurse Educator colleagues. However, as the Pharmacy—Nursing coordinator, she is now an intermediary between two very different disciplines. Cindy often feels oppressed by the volume of complaints from both the Pharmacy and Nursing departments. Furthermore, information technology intimidates Cindy. She often wishes she had the confidence and techno-savvy she witnesses in her two teenagers.

Information Systems Overview

The Santiago Health organization has had success in implementing information technology systems. In fact, Santiago was an early leader, implementing computerized physician order entry (CPOE) more than a decade ago. Santiago Health's leaders and their Marketing group like to boast that Santiago is a technology innovator, and they are anxious to add BPOC to the list of accomplishments that differentiate Santiago from its competitors.

Santiago Health has been able to outperform its peers in the healthcare market financially for many years. However, recent negative trends are worrying the president and CEO. A very large academic medical center nearby is simultaneously implementing CPOE as well as building a major new cardiac care center to compete with Santiago. Meanwhile, the case mix at the SCC shifted toward patients without health insurance when the state forced the closing of a small community hospital nearby. Finally, fiscal year performance is poor at Salty Waters Hospital, part of the Santiago Health system.

To date, the Santiago Health IS strategy has been to select "best of breed" solutions and to write custom interfaces to exchange data between them. This approach keeps the IS department busy updating and maintaining the interfaces and fixing broken links among the numerous disparate systems.

Implementing BPOC will require the Pharmacy department to replace, in its entirety, the antiquated Pharmacy information system. A gradual migration to a new Pharmacy system is not possible. Not only is this expensive, but it is also extremely disruptive to existing business processes. It will require new hardware, software, and even a new relationship with a different drug wholesaler. BPOC requires the reengineering and redefinition of many Pharmacy tasks and positions. Furthermore, there will be additional tasks, not the least of which is the repackaging of medications that arrive without bar codes.

The IS department is truly not concerned about the increase in hardware support for BPOC. However, additional requirements on Mr. Desco's group will be learning to install, operate, and maintain some unfamiliar hardware, as well as ordering and stocking new handheld BPOC units and their components. The IS department will also need to allocate resources for installing and testing the new BPOC application and its new server hardware. According to IS, the wireless local area network (LAN) is ready to go.

Complicating the BPOC implementation at Santiago Health is the fact that Santiago operates two smaller institutions, Camino Hospital and Salty Waters Hospital. Both are in nearby cities. Because of their small size, these two outlying hospitals rely on remote Pharmacy services provided by the Pharmacy department at the SCC from 5:00 p.m. in the evening until 7:00 a.m. the following morning are in nearby cities. Because of their small size, these two oulty-must provide a means to troubleshoot the BPOC system remotely for effective use at Camino and Salty Waters. No one at Santiago Health has formally addressed this issue to date.

The Problem

Several months ago, the Pharmacy department installed a software upgrade for the SCC automated dispensing machine (ADM) system. Communication broke down between the ADM vendor and Pharmacy. The vendor told Pharmacy that the new software would not affect the end users in Nursing. Assuming this to be true, Pharmacy chose a direct rollout of the new software version. On rollout day, and for several days after, irate nurses inundated Pharmacy with phone calls. The ADM user experience degraded after the software update and nurses had a difficult time getting medications. Unable to provide a quick solution, Pharmacy had no choice but to abandon the upgrade and return to the previous version of ADM software. At all levels, Nursing was annoyed with Pharmacy because of the insensitivity of implementing a significant ADM software change without warning.

From the Nursing point of view, they see Pharmacy as a driver for BPOC implementation. However, Pharmacy is being more careful with BPOC by considering its impact on staff nurses. Although it was outside of its purview, Pharmacy contacted both BPOC system vendors and handheld device vendors, and studied these products. Meanwhile, the implementation team at Santiago Health decided to go with the WowEm! Quick Check Bar Code Verifier. They chose this handheld device because it was fast, accurate, and it looked durable. The Pharmacy-Nursing coordinator, Cindy Marshall, especially appreciated that the WowEm! company offered 24/7 tech support and promised to ship a replacement device by overnight express if necessary.

A number of SCC staff members also attended a bar code implementation seminar to find out about any potential BPOC implementation problems. This trip included Jen Goodman, Rene Rousseau, Andrew Foor, and Sue Portal. Sue represented Nursing on behalf of Cindy Marshall who was unavailable. Through their discussions this multidisciplinary team came to recognize that although many healthcare organizations have applied information technology to parts of the medication use cycle, not one organization has successfully achieved a total information technology solution protecting patients from medication order (CPOE), to medication administration (BPOC), and to drug monitoring (Clinical Decision Support and the Electronic Health Record (EHR)). However, during the trip home from the seminar a clash erupted between Sue Portal and the others when Rene Rousseau commented that BPOC was so important that, "our nurses will just have to get used to it." Sue Portal returned to her Nursing unit quite defensive and angry about BPOC rollout plans at the SCC.

Dr Trubelli has recently learned that a consortium of major health insurance companies will require bar coding at point of care beginning in March of 2006. At that time these companies will expect 30% of all doses given to be verified using BPOC. By March of 2008, they will expect 90% BPOC compliance. These health insurance carriers are dealing with costs due to injuries from medication errors. This insurance company consortium intends to provide fiscal incentives for BPOC. Dr Trubelli is watching this development very carefully and has just set an organizational deadline of January 2006 for BPOC implementation at Santiago Health. When Kevin Dininger heard this news, his immediate response was, "It's not possible to implement this in only 13 months!" Sue Portal called Cindy Marshall to complain about the distancing of Nursing from discussions about the new deadline.

Main Issues

Pharmacy has a deadline to implement BPOC, yet those involved in the implementation come to the project with differing levels of knowledge about BPOC technology and differing awareness of the workflow impacts.

Communication, whether formal or informal, is absent or fragmented among the key players in Pharmacy, Nursing, and IS. Project success is dependent on effective communication within and among the groups involved.

Dr Trubelli's optimistic view of the project may not accurately reflect what other people in the organization are feeling. It is possible that, in terms of emotional intelligence, his self-motivation dominates his ability to empathize. Does his communication style cause others to feel uncomfortable in providing honest feedback? In any case, failure to see the potential risks and contrary opinions may lead him to advocate an unrealistically aggressive timeline for the program, whose failure will come as a complete surprise.

The IS leadership and the Desktop and Device services group may underestimate the challenges of implementing and supporting BPOC.

No other healthcare organization has implemented a comprehensive IS strategy to improve the entire medication use cycle. At Santiago, the combination of CPOE and BPOC with a planned EHR will be a significant advancement toward a more comprehensive medication safety system. However, while they think of themselves as groundbreakers, Santiago pharmacists are cognizant of the healthcare industry's scant history with BPOC and have much uncertainty about the rollout in their environment.

Nursing has no experience using this system and is unfamiliar with specific BPOC processes. Historical failures, such as the recent ADM software upgrade, will come to mind as BPOC arrives on the Nursing units. Perception plays a large role in acceptance.

Options with Pros and Cons

Option 1

Jen Goodman holds a team meeting with key players to discuss BPOC implementation and the new timeline set by Dr Trubelli.

Pros

It is essential to open the lines of communication and engage all stakeholders. Group efforts with the opportunity to present all sides will lead to buy-in from participants. Jen's staff and others in IS will become aware of concerns in Pharmacy and Nursing. Everyone has the opportunity to state concerns and resolve conflict about the project before implementation. It is particularly important to facilitate upward communication to Dr Trubelli, so that he is fully aware of progress as well as challenges faced by the stakeholders. The team may consider specific communication measures, such as a group email list, a periodic newsletter, or a project website, to encourage communication among the stakeholders.

Cons

Pharmacy, Nursing, and IS staff may not be aware or privy to all the possible problems that can arise during and after implementation. They must feel free to discuss questions, concerns, and criticisms in the formal meeting. Should conflict be irresolvable, the group may not reach a consensus. If the new deadline for implementation is unacceptable to all parties at this meeting, it may be a disturbing option for both Dr Trubelli and the Executive Management team.

Option 2

Consider a phased BPOC implementation strategy. Require bar code scanning at the bedside only for the most commonly prescribed medications. The first phase should not require additional packaging or handling of medications by the Pharmacy department. Once BPOC is functional, additional medications can gradually become a part of the BPOC system.

Pros

This option allows all affected groups to get a better sense of their workflow impacts without the burden of switching to a new system across the board. The old system and processes serve as a "safety net" in situations when the bar coding system fails. Groups may then have a role in examining the failures and solving BPOC problems. The trial period allows stakeholders to solicit feedback and refine processes before rolling out a total BPOC solution.

Cons

A staged approach requires support of two systems. In addition, it requires the nurse-users to manage and maintain two processes for drug administration. Studies of successful BPOC implementations have shown that 90% of medications need to be administered using the BPOC system in order to achieve the safety and efficiency gains that justify the investment in BPOC. If Nursing does not buy-in to BPOC from the start, it may tarnish the reputation of this technology and jeopardize expanded use of BPOC.

Option 3

Set up a test environment for staff to practice and learn the BPOC system in advance of the conversion to the new BPOC system and methods.

Pros

Staff gains confidence using the system before rollout. Various functional groups learn about each other's roles and tasks and have an opportunity to explain their particular requirements.

Cons

Test environments require additional resources (human, time, equipment, space) to gather and interpret results from users of the new system. Project management is necessary and this work may overwhelm current leaders or conflict with timelines for other projects. Test environments can be overly simplistic and therefore, poor representations of how the BPOC system will work with true clinical scenarios and large volumes of data.

Option 4

Extend the deadline for converting to BPOC or delay the start date for the project.

Pros

Staff may respond to additional time for familiarization and training. It also allows time to address key Pharmacy issues. Drug manufacturers and wholesalers planning to implement changes to their packaging and supply chains may have new systems ready in concert with new BPOC timelines at Santiago Health. This option may therefore reduce hospital costs incurred for repackaging and bar coding medications.

Cons

The main motivator for the BPOC initiative – dramatically decreasing the potential risk of medication errors – continues to exist during the extended timeline period. Many project management studies reveal that work tends to evolve closer to project start dates and end dates with lag time in the center. Moving the dates does not guarantee solid project management. Furthermore, organizationally this course would involve a showdown between the high-level leadership and operational managers in Pharmacy and Nursing. The rift created could jeopardize the entire BPOC project.

Question

Which option would you choose and why?

Key Stakeholders for BPOC Planning and Implementation

1. Dr Trubelli, MD, is the Medical Director for IS at Santiago Health. He formerly held positions as the Chairman of Pediatrics and Medical Director for the Neonatal Intensive Care Unit. He believes BPOC will face little resistance and facilitate workflow. Dr Trubelli has a special interest in using bar coding to identify blood products and breast milk.

2. Rene Rousseau, RPh, is the Clinical Liaison for Santiago Health's implementation of Project Genesis. This encompasses system wide programs including the migration to Cerner Millennium. Rene does not fit neatly into the organizational chart. He is on loan from other areas.

3. Kevin Dininger, RPh, is the Service Delivery Leader (SDL) and Operations Manager for Pharmacy Services at Santiago Health. Andrew Foor, RPh, the Pharmacy Informatics Coordinator reports directly to Kevin. Kevin cites many hindrances to Pharmacy workflow with the BPOC project. He is very concerned about Nursing processes and fostering collaboration in advance of the BPOC implementation.

4. Andrew Foor, RPh, has dual roles as the Pharmacy Informatics Coordinator and as a Staff Pharmacist. Andrew has a big picture view of BPOC, understanding technological, organizational, and process impacts. He, like Cindy and Jen, has concerns about the project timeline. He emphasizes meeting educational needs in advance of implementation.

5. Cindy Marshall, RN is the Pharmacy/Nursing Coordinator. It is her job to bring the Pharmacy and Nursing departments together on a variety of patient care issues. Like Andrew, she reports to the Pharmacy Operations Manager, Mr. Dininger. She is cognizant of the inherent workflow demands of nurses and will be the recipient of both praise and criticism when BPOC begins. Cindy has a firm grasp of the project timelines and educational needs for Nursing.

6. Carl Desco is an IS Manager in the data processing & desktop systems division. Carl will be responsible for the servers and other IT infrastructure necessary to operate the bar coding system. He is isolated from the organizational issues. Carl anticipates an increased demand for hardware support during the first month of BPOC but then expects to return to business as usual.

7. Jen Goodman is a Regional Information Services Director. Jen was promoted recently and she embraces technology solutions, including BPOC, with a positive demeanor. She expresses concern about hardware and software issues with a tendency to minimize the organizational impacts expressed by Pharmacy and Nursing. Jen is a bit uneasy about the date milestones but overall she is highly committed to the BPOC project. Jen has connections at the highest levels of Santiago Health leadership. She exhibits strong leadership in many ways. She is a particularly good listener while she smartly defends the view from the executive suites at Santiago Health without hesitation.

8. Sally Portal, RN, is a unit nurse and will be one of the first users of the BPOC system. Like many nurses, she has heard the term BPOC but has no in-depth knowledge of the project.

7
Different Sides of the Story

Allison B. McCoy

Introduction

Providing effective decision support to physicians in care provider order entry (CPOE) systems is a recurring challenge for informatics staff. Reminders or alerts displayed to providers easily convey knowledge to assist with patient encounters, often reducing errors in patient care.[1,2] However, studies show that providers may develop "alert fatigue" and ignore the alerts and reminders displayed in computer systems. A high rate of nonserious, irrelevant, and repeated alerts most often contributes to alert fatigue among providers.[1] The ability to appropriately alert providers, at the right time, with the correct type of support, and at an appropriate level of intrusiveness, is critical in the reduction of alert fatigue and ultimately in the success of decision support systems in improving quality and safety of patient care.[2]

The Location

Valley Regional Medical Center (VRMC) is a 1,000-bed academic tertiary care facility in the central region of the US. The adult medical intensive care unit (MICU) is a 26-bed general medicine intensive care unit. Providers at VRMC use a locally developed and maintained CPOE system and electronic medical record (EMR) with multiple levels of decision support. Some forms of decision support include dose guidance at the order construction phase and pharmacy alerts for drug–drug and drug-allergy interactions. Pharmacy alerts appear as pop-ups initially and later as persistent text in an order summary screen panel.

The Actors

Two teams of providers care for the patients in the MICU. Each team consists of an attending physician along with one or more fellows, residents, interns, and medical students, and optionally a dietician. Additionally, librarians may round with the team to follow up with answers to in-depth research questions that may benefit individual patients.

L. Einbinder et al. (eds.), *Transforming Health Care Through Information:*
Case Studies, Health Informatics, DOI 10.1007/978-1-4419-0269-6_7,
© Springer Science+Business Media, LLC 2010

The Story

On a typical day, provider teams meet together to make rounds on the patients. On average, the team cares for 8–10 patients daily. Each provider carries a printed current medications and results rounding sheet for each patient. This sheet contains important information about the patient, including alerts such as potential drug interaction warnings. Each of the fellows, residents, interns, and medical students visits the patient prior to the rounds. The intern is responsible for reporting each patient's history and current status to the attending physician and the team during the rounds. In addition, another team member uses a portable clinical workstation to access the EMR, CPOE, and other systems during the rounds. After seeing each patient, the team member will enter orders directly into the CPOE system, where he or she may see decision support alerts. After the team has seen all the assigned patients, the fellows, residents, and interns will meet separately to modify and enter final orders on the patients, again using the CPOE system and possibly viewing alerts.

When asked, MICU providers respond favorably toward decision support alerts. One provider comments that "The pop-ups are helpful and usually help me remember information I might have overlooked." Another provider agrees that the alerts are beneficial, but admits to occasionally ignoring or quickly overriding alerts if they are repetitive or irrelevant.

Direct observations and data from system usage logs tell a different side of the story. During the observations, providers tended to skim alert text and frequently override warnings. One provider, when too quickly trying to complete a pop-up form, received multiple errors for missing required fields before he was able to submit the data. When asked about the persistent pharmacy alert text, another provider admits to never noticing the messages. Usage logs for the CPOE system obtained by informatics staff backup these observations; providers override a majority of displayed pop-up pharmacy alerts. Also, logs show that providers almost never click links to display additional advice. Despite their belief that they utilize the provided decision support, in practice, providers pay little attention to most alerts.

Summary/Questions

1. Providers and informatics staff often see different sides of the decision support alert story. While both groups agree on the benefits that alerts may offer, in practice, providers more often ignore alerts than utilize the information provided.
2. Should informatics staff devote time and effort to developing the alert support if providers disregard the advice?
3. How can informatics staff develop decision support alerts that providers are willing to utilize?
4. Should informatics staff or providers be responsible for preventing the development of alert fatigue?
5. Can the problem be solved, or will providers continue to disregard even the best system?

References

1. Van der Sijs H, Aarts J, Vulto A, Berg M. Overriding of drug safety alerts in computerized physician order entry. *J Am Med Inform Assoc*. 2006;13:138-147.
2. Miller RA, Waitman LR, Chen S, Rosenbloom ST. The anatomy of decision support during inpatient care provider order entry (CPOE): empirical observations from a decade of CPOE experience at Vanderbilt. *J Biomed Inform*. 2005;38(6):469-485.

8
Barcode Medication Administration Implementation in the FIAT Health System

LINDA CHAN, WILLIAM GREELEY, DON KLINGEN, BRIAN MACHADO, MICHAEL PADULA, JOHN SUM, and ANGELA VACCA

Introduction

"Don't you see? This won't make a difference in the long run," pleaded Dr. Target, the Medical Director of Information Services.

Dr. Target was attending a process review meeting and could tell she was not convincing anyone. She was at a root cause analysis meeting because of a medication error that she knew could have been prevented.

A physician had correctly written for 10 units of insulin to be given to a patient following correct JCAHO protocol and writing the number 10 without a trailing zero as well as the word "units" in clear legible writing.

Unfortunately, the unit clerk erroneously transcribed the order as 100 units to the paper Medication Administration Record (MAR). The patient consequently received 10 times the intended dose of insulin.

Dr. Target continued, "Have you ever been on the floors and seen all the tasks the clerks have to juggle? When a physician writes an order, the clerks must fax it to the pharmacy and then transcribe the medication order to the paper MAR. The person with the least clinical knowledge is responsible for setting up the patient's MAR. Do you realize that while they are doing this, they are also answering the phone, jockeying for access to the chart and answering questions. It's a wonder that this didn't happen sooner."

"While you may feel disciplining her is the right thing to do, I highly doubt we have done anything to prevent this from happening again" Dr. Target concluded.

The chairman of the committee replied, "I know where you are going with this. You want to make a pitch for the bar coded medication project. Don't tell us that one of your computer systems could have prevented this. We've heard that before… Is this as good as the electronic nursing documentation system your group tried to implement at the other hospital and failed? This clerk made a costly mistake and needs to be held accountable."

Dr. Target was facing an uphill battle and she knew it. On the one hand the CIO, Mr. Dewy Yesterday, declared that FIAT health system would go live with bar coded medication administration (BCMA) within the next year. On the other hand, Dr. Target had significant resistance from groups like these.

L. Einbinder et al. (eds.), *Transforming Health Care Through Information: Case Studies*, Health Informatics, DOI 10.1007/978-1-4419-0269-6_8, © Springer Science+Business Media, LLC 2010

The business and strategy reasons for implementing BCMA were compelling. FIAT health system had just upgraded its enterprise laboratory and pharmacy systems. These were the last of the infrastructure to be put in place to allow for next level applications such as BCMA and eventually computerized physician order entry. BCMA was one more step of FIAT health system's pursuit of its vision of "Clinical Transformation" from paper to electronic systems. In addition, the health system from the neighboring county was starting to make in-roads and compete in FIATs catchment area. The CIO felt the need to compete from a technology standpoint.

However, for an equal number of reasons, the environment for implementing such a system was hostile. The nursing and pharmacy departments,which were expected to implement and adopt it, had little input for selecting the system yet. The medication workflow for nursing and pharmacy had not been examined yet. Logistically, the pharmacy department did not have the capacity or equipment to package medications from multidose vials into single-dose packages.

There was also the past history of information technology implementations at FIAT health system that had to be addressed. FIAT health care is a loosely federated health care system with three community hospitals and one tertiary care hospital. Previously, all the information system needs were outsourced. Eight years ago, the CIO brought all information system departments in-house and upgraded the network infrastructure. He then set about an aggressive plan of "Clinical Transformation" to convert FIAT health care from a paper based to an electronic process.

Things were going well until they attempted to implement electronic nursing documentation in two of the community hospitals. The system used for the documentation was an old green screen/light pen DOS-based system. Physicians at one of the community put up so much resistance to the project that further progress was halted until the system could be updated to a more modern web-based look and feel.

Against this backdrop, Dr. Target was trying to lead the charge for BCMA. Realizing the political and implementation challenges, she decided to get some outside help to evaluate the best plan for going forward.

Dr. Target enlisted the help of "Team Barcode" to assess her organization and look for the best strategy to implement BCMA.

Methods

Dr. Target called upon a group of individuals currently enrolled at OHSU in the informatics program to discuss the situation at FIAT. She wanted to seek a sounding board to validate issues and utilize their knowledge to strategize how to move forward with the project.

In order to assess the situation of FIAT health systems, "Team Barcode" interviewed key stakeholders and the implementation team, and also sought to develop a survey tool to examine the organization's readiness for BCMA. A literature search revealed a standardized survey tool developed by a coalition group of the American Hospital Association, Health Research and Education Trust, and the Institute for Safe Medication Practice entitled "Readiness Assessment for a Bedside Bar-Coded Drug Administration System".[1]

The readiness assessment survey encompasses 135 items divided into nine distinct elements related to successful implementation of BCMA. Each item is scored based on that item being: (a) fully implemented, (b) partially implemented, or (c) not implemented.

Several of these items are felt to be prerequisites that must be in place before BCMA can be implemented, while others are facilitators that will simply make it easier to implement BCMA.

In order to get an organization-wide view, the survey was administered to eight senior leadership members of FIAT and front line staff. Among the senior leadership, the Vice President of Quality and Safety was unable to complete the survey and is left out of this report. In total, almost all of the survey questions were answered completely and compiled in this report. The exceptions were the CIO who answered less than one quarter of the questions, and the local hospital pharmacist who answered less than two thirds of the questions.

A nursing survey was also performed that was based partly on the readiness assessment survey, and also on literature regarding nursing satisfaction with medication administration (the MAS–NAS scale).[2] The survey consisted of 19 questions that encompassed individual, group, and organization issues. Thirty nurses responded to the questionnaire, comprising a representative sample of nurses on the general medicine wards. A cross survey analysis was also performed.

Results

BCMA Readiness Survey Results

The following is the summary of the management survey findings:

Drug Labeling, Packaging, and Nomenclature
The packaging and labeling of drugs are not ready for BCMA. There are concerns on the availability of unit-dose drug packages and the capability to print bar code labels for pharmacy-prepared, patient-specific unit-dose medication.

Drug Standardization, Storage, and Distribution
Nursing and pharmacy have different views on drug standardization and how to handle exceptional drug processes.

Environmental Factors
The physical environment of both pharmacy and nursing is not yet ready to handle the extra hardware necessary to implement BCMA. There are different views as to whether pharmacy and nursing follow a consistent workflow process.

Patient Information
Practical and technical aspects of the patient identification work flow are not well established.

Drug Information
Despite the impending implementation, little consideration has been given to the selection of pharmacy products or vendors that are compatible with bar coding. It has not impacted current formulary decisions.

Communication of Drug Orders and Other Drug Information
The MAR is not well unified across the system for all medications.

Staff Competency and Education
In general, competency in information technology is felt to be high at FIAT. However, education of front line clinical staff in BCMA technology is sorely lack-

ing. Plans for such training, and for dealing with technical failure have also not been implemented and need to be done.

Patient Education
Patient education seems to be relatively lacking as patients and patient groups have been left out of BCMA plans at FIAT health system.

Quality Processes and Risk Management
Several deficiencies in leadership were recognized including: effective communication of BCMA as part of the overall strategic plan, commitment to allocate sufficient resources, proper alignment of BCMA with other parts of the hospital system and government regulations, and a lack of involvement of front line nurses and pharmacists in planning. It is also not clear that FIAT has compiled teams to work together to support technology issues, and BCMA issues in particular.

Safety and medical errors are seen by leadership as important issues that should not be used in a punitive fashion. However, there appears to be some underlying anxiety as "off the record" discussions are not promoted, and pharmacy actually feels that such feedback mechanisms are not in place at all. Also, while senior management reports a strong interest in medication safety, the pharmacy does not believe this to be the case.

Nursing Survey Results

The following is a summary of the Nursing survey findings:

The nursing staff felt confident that BCMA would enhance the safe and efficient delivery of patient care without having any adverse affect on their role. They also reported foreseeing that patients would feel safer knowing that BCMA was being used.

The survey tool demonstrated several concerns as well. Training and education as well as the rationale for implementing BCMA and its impact on nursing work flow were rated low. The perceived lack of nursing involvement in BCMA planning and implementation was also noted. The survey identified a lack of awareness of who the nursing and pharmacy leaders/champions of this new initiative were. Finally, the nursing staff felt a lack of awareness of FIATs overall IT strategy.

Cross-Survey Results

Several of the questions from the BCMA readiness survey mapped directly to the Nursing survey. Overall, both leadership and the nurses felt that the strategic reason for BCMA and its impact on workflow had not been explained to nursing. They both felt that nurses were not involved in the planning for the implementation of the BCMA. On the positive side, both felt that the organization had success and experience in integrating and interfacing various information systems.

With regards to the health system senior leadership's view of BCMA, nursing felt that management was supportive of the project, whereas there was disagreement amongst the leadership on this issue.

Access to supportive systems for medication administration was also a point of discord: nursing felt they had the tools necessary whereas the leadership surveys felt there could be more to be done.

Nurses were either generally neutral or agreed that they could discuss medication errors, near misses or barriers to medication administration with leadership. This raises some question as to whether a culture of candor truly exists at FIAT. One would think that if such a culture were in place, there would be a more positive response on this issue. Assessment of the leadership showed that they did not feel that these communication pathways were fully implemented.

Analysis and Recommendations

On the basis of survey results, interviews, and understanding of the FIAT culture, the following themes for analysis and recommendations were developed:

Strategic Planning

It seems that the management of FIAT has adopted a quasi-imitation strategy in terms of the BCMA initiative. Clearly there is motivation to demonstrate innovation in an extremely cost efficient manner that is driven by market dynamics. However, there appears to be no demonstrable high-level strategic plan containing a tactical implementation outline with clear milestones – one of which is BCMA.

Given that the organization has embarked on a tactical implementation without fully defining and elaborating the overall strategic plan, the following are our recommendations for creating a sustainable plan.

The Board and Senior Management will need to create a series of short term committees each charged with a specific aspect of the strategic vision. Some suggested committees are:

A Marketing and Business Development Committee which is tasked with focusing its efforts on identifying the geographic sections of the service area that are out of the immediate primary service area and where partnership strategies with medical groups etc. should be pursued to manage clinical program and partnership development. Maintenance of a health care leadership position in the community requires leadership in the application of new clinical technologies, with perhaps expertise in specific niches, and excellence in the delivery of specialty care.

A Clinical Effectiveness Initiative Committee which is to focus on identifying options for achieving greater clinical and operational efficiencies and increasing marketplace competitiveness. This would roll up well under a quality program.

An Information Technology Strategic Planning Committee which would be responsible for developing a vision for future information technology capabilities that is critical to keeping the health system at the forefront in clinical information technology. This committee would have to account for the recommendations of the prior committees and develop the IT strategic vision to complement those recommendations. Additionally, the committee would also need to work closely with finance and the facilities departments to ensure that the normal operational process of maintenance and replacement of existing and aging technology is done in conjunction with the IT plan to allow for effective utilization of scarce capital dollars. This structure will help FIAT continue to plan developments in information technology concomitant with infrastructure replacement, with a focus on meeting immediate needs while also planning the hospital of the future.

To that end the IT Strategic Planning Committee should develop an exhaustive list of the current state of technology at each of the four sites. Any common platform should be leveraged as a spring-board to build upon. Facilities and biomedical engineering should bring a list of all equipment with any tie-in to IT. That list should have the purchase date of the asset together with expected life and replacement date. These lists need to be compiled into a master list which also combines routine capital requests from the clinical departments. The committee should then review the entire compilation and come up with a composite list of items that have clinical and strategic implications over 1-, 3-, 5- and 10-year horizons. The list should also have approximate costs and implementation timelines to ensure adequate planning for lead times.

Given the complexity of the planning process, we would suggest that the list be given to the Board and each of the subcommittees to do a forced ranking of priorities. The final ranked lists should then be compared to come up with a common list of items than can be further fleshed out for the final approval of the board. It is also imperative that critical stakeholders be involved in developing an implementation plan of the tactical strategies put down by the management team.

Operationally, the framework as outlined by Davis and Adams[3] in their article in the *Journal of Healthcare Financial Management* seems pertinent:

1. Recognize how differently your organization may have to operate during the planning horizon. Possibly develop an annual plan, a longer-term (such as 3 years) plan, and even a longer-term perspective such as a strategic vision supported by critical assumptions. Evaluate strategic alternatives and proposals in light of all three time frames.
2. Make sure your longer-term plan and strategic vision are detailed enough to frame your organization's IT strategy. For example, it is not enough to simply state that improving clinical quality is a goal; it is important to understand what the organization is doing to improve clinical quality and how IT can help.
3. Frame the planning effort with guardrails – particularly financial guardrails. For example, what is the capital or operating limits to which the organization and the IT-related spending must adhere?
4. Ask the IT people to speak the language of your business rather than "techno-speak." Expect strategic alternatives, and agree on a set of criteria to evaluate those alternatives.
5. Examine technologies such as portals and analytics tools to extend the use of your data to enable true business value through enhanced information access, sharing, and analysis.
6. Ensure that your technology strategy is based on open technology standards and enables the use of reusable assets to leverage existing technology (e.g., service-oriented architecture).

As you begin your next strategic IT planning process, envision an IT-enabled organization operating in a much different healthcare environment – one that is moving toward being more patient-centric, value-based, accountable, affordable, and sustainable.

Leadership – Integration of the Clinical and Technological Aspects

Leadership is defined as the ability to influence a group towards the achievement of a vision or a set of goals.[4] It is, therefore clear that leaders and leadership must play a critical role in managing technological change[5] like the institution of a BCMA. There are both organizational as well as personal factors that are important in achieving effective leadership which will then lead to successful technological change. There must also be a good match between the leadership style and stage of organizational growth.[4,6] These factors within FIAT health system must be analyzed to understand the leadership issue, and possible solutions/improvements.

For FIAT health system, one of the major organizational factors to affect leadership includes the organizational legitimization of leaders, which is important to avoid a leadership vacuum.[7] In the case of FIAT, there is a Medical Director of IS (effectively a CMIO), but without formal power or a clearly expressed scope of management. It is well known that one of the strongest barriers to CMIO effectiveness is a lack of support or access to senior management.[8,9] Without the strong backing of senior leadership, informatics leaders can lose credibility and projects will flounder.[10]

Personal leadership factors are also important. Eight behavior-knowledge sets of leadership success in health informatics have been outlined, with a high score required on all factors.[7] The CIO, one of the most important key leaders in the BCMA initiative, is rated on this inventory in Table 8.1. There are clearly some areas that need improvement for successful change to be established. The CIO may have a vision for the organization, but it has not been effectively communicated. It is not clear if the past nursing documentation failure has been appreciated, and the CIO has not empowered his followers.

The organizational structure of FIAT also impacts leadership style. FIAT is more along the lines of a Stage 2 organization as described by Lorenzi and Riley.[7] There are very distinct functional areas such as nursing, information technology, pharmacy, etc. Unfortunately, this stage is often marked by lower motivation and commitment, and employees usually do not see the big picture very well. Politically, FIAT is also more along the model of "Technocratic Utopianism" where the CIO is from the information technology industry, and believes more that the technology itself will provide the answers to every information problem.[7] This particular organizational structure may require a leader who is of more high task, low relations (whip cracker), and is more reactive than proactive. In the case of FIAT, the CIO seems to be more low task and low people, and is perhaps more willing to abdicate some of his responsibilities. This may not be a good leader/organizational stage fit.

Recommendations Regarding Leadership

Creation and appointment of a full-time formal CMIO position with formal power and authority and with well-defined responsibilities. To be effective, the CMIO must have access to adequate resources and be made a senior member of the executive team with full support from upper management. This person should also possess strong interpersonal and communication skills, and have the respect of the medical staff.[8,9]

The CIO will need to work to correct some of the deficiencies seen in Table 8.1. This can be accomplished by leadership training[11] and coaching in emotional intelligence.[6] This may help to create a better leader/organizational fit.

The CIO must work within the organization to create a future vision and also effectively communicate that vision and the IT goals to the organization. The CIO will need to learn to adjust leadership style to the stage of the organization, and adapt an affiliate style of leadership in order to develop and empower his subordinates, especially the CMIO and other managers.[12] Leading nursing, pharmacy, and others with an affiliate style will improve organizational climate and communication.

TABLE 8.1   Inventory of Behavior Knowledge Set

Behavior knowledge set	Low	←---→>	High
Understands the big picture in both health care and informatics, and has established a vision to encompass the big picture		X	
Has established clear and focused goals	X		
Has identified and assessed different situations and effectively used the appropriate leadership style(s)		X	
Has learned from past successes and failures	X		
Has developed and empowered people	X		
Communicates clearly	X		
Has a positive self-esteem			X
Understands and uses power			X

The CIO should use his knowledge of power to facilitate action and movement towards the BCMA vision. This may include developing cross functional teams, encouraging a culture of change, and supporting strategic planning. Part of this developmental process may also include acknowledging the past IT nursing documentation failure, learning from this failure, and translating this to the entire organization.[7]

The CIO should better assess the introduction of health information technology into their social, work and technical environments. The CIO should not assume that these implementations are merely a technology installation.

Project Management

The process of FIATs BCMA implementation lacks important principles fundamental to managing the project successfully. The project was initiated with inadequate involvement of the stakeholders, and many critical details necessary for a comprehensive project plan are lacking.

In order to attempt to optimize this project in progress, it would be best to more precisely establish the scope and deliverables of the project. The scope and deliverables should be developed with the input of IT, nursing and pharmacy representatives. Project-level performance measures will need to be identified to ensure that the objectives of the program are achieved. Project scope should then be determined so that clarity is obtained on what BCMA will include and not include.

With the scope established, the key participants for input and communication will be more readily apparent. It is telling that the Vice President of Patient Safety and Quality was unaware of the project, while safety is likely one of the foremost objectives of the BCMA implementation. Key leaders need to be identified and contacted for their input and to help communicate the project scope.

To flesh out the details of the project plan, techniques such as a work breakdown structure should be employed to fully identify each of the steps and deliverables in the project.[13] It is important that the deliverables be specific, measurable, realistic and timely. This work plan needs to have a well established time line with specific check points to monitor the progress. Ownership and accountability for each process step needs to be established. It is important to identify the dependencies (i.e. points in the process which depend upon completion of a prior step) for each deliverable.[14]

In regards to pharmacy, implications of BCMA need to be considered in establishing which drugs are on the formulary and how such drugs are purchased and packaged. Contingency plans should also be delineated for scenarios in which the system is unable to function as designed and workflows need to be restructured.

A project is dependent on the resources which support it. Proper allocation of financial resources along with the appropriate personnel is essential in order to keep the project afloat. Detailed accounting of the project steps should help to keep such costs in a more tangible perspective. The project plan should address the following areas:

- Project governance should be clearly defined with everyone involved understanding their roles and responsibilities.
- Executive Sponsors should support the program in a consistent and visible way.
- A cost model will be required for the project and will include both operational and technical costs
- Appropriate resources should be assigned to the project to ensure the successful outcome of the objectives for the project.
- Funding and resources should be adequate to meet the needs of the project.
- Project teams should be created and notified of their participation on the project as a part of the process for chartering a new project.
- An agreed-upon organizational change management approach should be implemented for the project.
- Training will be required for all employees who will be impacted by the BCMA implementation.
- Support: Adequate tools including hardware and software will be available for all areas of the enterprise necessary to support the project.
- Interfaces: The scope of interface development, execution, procurement should be assessed.
- Risk: During the startup phase of the project, risks will be identified and mitigation strategies developed. This process will be ongoing and will require updated assessments to evaluate the status of the identified risks as well as any potential new risks.
- Communications: Detailed communication plans defining what information should be communicated with whom and how often should be developed in advance to make sure proper and consistent communication is present throughout the project.

Introduction of Technology into Workflow

It is clear that workflow has not been carefully looked at throughout the implementation and that the CIO expects technology to fix the current process problems. Massaro,[15] in his article, indicates that IT cannot fix problems it did not create and that technology can accentuate existing problems by diverting attention from the root causes and fundamental issues involved. In order to predict the impact that implementation of a new technology, such as BCMA, will have on nursing and pharmacy workflow, it is imperative that the workflow of the existing system is clearly understood. Neglecting a thorough workflow analysis could result in unanticipated and undesired consequences. These unintended consequences flow not from technological malfunctions, but from the interaction of technology with the existing workflow of the end user, and may have impacts that undermine patient care in immediate ways, such as the creation of new types of medical errors and, more indirectly, a negative impact on employee motivation.

To examine workflow, many studies have suggested direct observations and interviews of end users using the system. End users should be deeply involved in the project planning and implementation phases. Additionally, techniques such as simulation during the design phase can be used to gather information and design future workflow.

One of the most notorious unintended consequences of implementing technology without giving enough attention to workflow is workarounds. Workarounds occur when users "engage in problem-solving behaviors that involve bypassing new technology or adapting a work process so as to minimize disruption in work flow."[16] Workarounds are often used as a result of nursing frustration. Examples include ignoring system alerts, affixing patient ID barcodes (which are intended to appear on patient ID bracelets) to something other than the patient for ease of access, and scanning multiple patients' medications at the same time.

While undesirable, workarounds should not be neglected and can be viewed as opportunities for learning and improvement. The extent that workarounds persist should be used as a tool to inform system enhancement. Therefore, FIAT should perform a workflow analysis and adopt a feedback process that is iterative and analyzes the actual postimplementation experience of the end user through qualitative and quantitative methods. FIAT can thereby examine workarounds and use it as a tool in the design of a successful BCMA system.

Culture of Change

Barcode medication administration creates a significant change in the workflow and processes for many. In order for change of this type to last and be successful, the organization must first create a culture that is open to change. Such a culture is characterized by open and honest communication among leaders and employees, empowered employees, innovation, and sharing of knowledge.[17,18]

The survey analysis reveals that the culture in this organization is not strongly identified as encouraging trust and open communication. Unless there is a supportive and trusting culture, true issues cannot not be uncovered, which may intensify the resistance to change.

Frontline workers are also not directly involved in the planning of their workflow changes giving them a sense that decisions are forced upon them which often increases resistance to the change. Lastly, knowledge such as the organization's strategic plan, available current and future technology, and data on medication errors, is not commonly shared vertically (across all levels of employees) or horizontally (across different functional groups) in the organization. Sharing knowledge can enhance unity, promote diverse opinions on problem-solving, and avoid duplicate efforts.

Effective leadership has frequently been linked to leading changes.[19-22] Leaders often become an anchor and model for employees in times of change and ambiguity. As a result, leaders must maintain a positive attitude and be actively engaged in both planning and implementation of change. Organizational leadership such as the CEO, VPs, and department chairs must be committed to support change and integrate change efforts into the organization's overall strategic planning. There should also be key change leaders, such as local nursing and pharmacy directors, who are responsible for managing and implementing change initiatives and they should possess the ability to articulate the organization's vision, have the necessary formal and informal power to lead change, be flexible, be knowledgeable, and be able to handle resistance.[19] Leaders should also emphasize on the importance of spending time on problem identification and analysis, knowledge transfer, and reflective post-audits. When people in power demonstrate through their own behavior willingness to entertain alternative points of view, employees are more confident in offering new ideas and options.[23]

Organization's structure may also need to be redesigned, for example, to be more organic and flat so that employees can be empowered to make changes and to enhance vertical communications. A matrix reporting structure may also help break down boundaries between traditionally isolated functional departments. In addition, a project steering committee should be set up to update and monitor project progress, share information with key stakeholders and the rest of the organization, and make project decisions with the right authorities. This committee will enhance knowledge sharing, promote cross-function collaboration, monitor the progress and direction of the project, and acquire the appropriate buy-in and support. The project steering committee should include members of other strategic planning committees as suggested above in the strategic planning section.

Lastly, until new behaviors become the social norm they are subject to degradation.[24] Reinforcement can help recognize and confirm progress. The organization can reinforce innovative and open culture by rewarding people who are willing to identify broken processes and those who take chances to show that providing constructive criticisms, admitting failures, and taking risks are all desirable traits.[18] Furthermore, human resource may be involved to hire and promote those who possess these traits and those with values that would be congruent with the desired change.[25]

Conclusion

The analysis of FIAT outlines many requirements that should be implemented either prior to or as part of the BCMA project. First, the organizational structure should be reorganized and improvements in leadership need to be instituted in order to create the proper environment for technological change. Next, an organization-wide strategic plan should be adopted and data should be gathered from all levels of the organization. Communication channels need to be improved and cross functional teams need to be promoted to encourage innovation, trust, and improve the planning process. With this, a well designed project management and portfolio management system needs to be adopted with strict assessment of quality. From all of this should then be a natural flow towards a culture of change that is more likely to adapt new technology like BCMA.

Strategy, planning, communication, and logistics aside, the root issue at FIAT health system is that BCMA is not a technology project. Instead, it is a people and process project that touches many departments and workflows within the hospital. In order for the hardware and software to succeed a lot of attention needs to be spent on the "wetware" by getting the appropriate people to the table to examine the workflow and processes. Otherwise, Dr. Target will be attending another root cause analysis meeting for the same issue, but this time it could be due to a computer error.

In closing, "Team Barcode" enjoyed the opportunity to work with Dr. Target on this project. Outside of the need to produce a report for Dr. Target, each member of the team felt they were able to explore an issue of personal interest and further develop the principles they learned at OHSU.

References

1. Readiness Assessment for a Bedside Bar-Coded Drug Administration System. American Hospital Association, Health Research & Educational Trust, and the Institute for Safe Medication Practices. Chicago, IL. http://www.medpathways.info/medpathways/tools/content/3_2.pdf; 2002. Accessed 18.05.08.

2. Hurley AC, Lancaster DR, Hayes J, et al. The medication administration system-nurses assessment of satisfaction (MAS-NAS) scale. *J Nurs Scholarsh*. 2006;38:298-300.

3. Davis D, Adams J. IT strategic planning: what healthcare CFOs should know. *J Healthc Financ Manage*. 2007;61(11):100-102, 104.

4. Robbins SP, Judges TA. *Organizational Behavior*. 12th ed. Pearson Prentice Hall: Saddle River, NJ; 2007:402.

5. Lorenzi NM, Riley RT. *Managing Technological Change: Organizational Aspects of Health Informatics*. 2nd ed. New York, NY: Springer; 2003:45-58.

6. Goleman D. Leadership that gets results. *Harv Bus Rev*. 2000;78(2):78-90.

7. Lorenzi NM, Riley RT. pp. 45-58.

8. Runy LA. The changing role of the CMIO. *Hosp Health Netw*. 2008;82(2):37-42.

9. Shaffer VL. Evolving Organization Needs and the Role of CMIO, AMDIS-Gartner Survey Findings. Available from the AMDIS website: http://www.amdis.org/2007%20AMDIS%20Gartner%20Survey.pdf; 2007. Accessed 11.05.08.

10. Lorenzi NM, Riley RT. p. 210.

11. Robbins SP, Judges TA. pp. 456-457.

12. Goleman D. pp. 78-90.

13. Project Management Institute. *Project Management Institute Practice Standard for Work Breakdown Structures*. 2nd ed. Newtown Square, PA: Project Management Institute; 2006:11-18.

14. Lientz BP, Rea KP. *Project Management for the 21st Century*. New York, NY: Academic Press; 2001:69-75.

15. Massaro TA. Introducing physician order entry at a major academic medical center: impact on organizational culture and behavior. *Acad Med*. 1993;68(1):20-25.

16. Vogelsmeier AA, Halbesleben JR, Scott-Cawiezell JR. pp. 114-119.

17. MacPhee M. Strategies and tools for managing change. *JONA*. 2007;37(9):405-413.

18. Robbins SP, Judge TA. *Organizational Behavior*. 12th ed. Upper Saddle River, NJ: Prentice-Hall; 2007.

19. Lorenzi NM, Riley RT. *Managing Technological Change: Organizational Aspects of Health Informatics*. 2nd ed. New York: Springer; 2004.

20. White A. Change strategies make for smooth transitions. *Nurs Manage*. 2004;35(2):49-52.

21. Herold DM, Fedor DB, Cadwell S, Liu Y. The effects of transformational and change leadership on employees' commitment to a change: a multilevel study. *J Appl Psycho*. 2008;93(2):346-357.

22. Luo JS, Hilty DM, Worley LL, Yager J. Considerations in change management related to technology. *Acad Psychiatry*. 2006;30(6):465-469.

23. Stinson L, Pearson D, Lucas B. Developing a learning culture: twelve tips for individuals, teams and organizations. *Med Teach*. 2006;28(4):309-312.

24. Kotter J. Leading change: why transformation efforts fail. *Harv Bus Rev*. 1995;73(2):59-67.

25. Salmond SW. Managing the human side of change. *Orthop Nurs*. 1998;17(5):38-51.

9
H.I.T. or Miss

James McCormack, Bimal R. Desai, Jennifer Garvin,
Randal Hamric, Kirk Lalwani, Andi Lushaj, Alexey Panchenko,
Deborah Quitmeyer, and JoAnna M. Vanderhoef

As hospitals become more electronic, smooth hospital operations become increasingly dependent on information systems. The following drama provides three perspectives on a series of HIT-related problems that occurred in a "model" IT-intensive hospital of the future.

Emily's Story

Emily sat down at her desk and picked up the red file folder labeled "Adverse Event Report." She had already heard about the incident last week with an ER patient, Mary Smith, who had suffered a severe drug reaction after being admitted to 3 West for pneumonia. Part of what bothered her was that after 15 years of service, the nurse involved had just resigned, claiming that a series of computer problems had led to Mary's near fatal reaction.

Like many health systems, Highland had spent millions of dollars on information systems intended to prevent the very problems that Mary and her family experienced that night. Something had gone terribly wrong, and Emily needed to report back the next day to the hospital quality assurance committee. Emily walked into the information services department and searched through the maze of cubicles to find Steven, the IT analyst who had been assigned by the CIO to help her with her investigation. "Hi, Steven, I'm Emily from Risk Management." she said, "Can I ask you a few questions about what happened last Thursday night?" Steven pulled up a chair for Emily, and cleared off a corner of his desk for her, moving aside vendor gadgets and knickknacks gathered during years of IT conferences. As she and Steven talked through the events, starting with Mary's admission to the ER through to her reaction to the drug in 3 West, one thing became clear – no single computer problem was to be blamed. Instead, a series of "glitches" almost led to a fatal medication error and to the resulting stack of incident reports in the red folder. Things started to go wrong when Dr. Kirk Lobson, a fixture at Highland and the chair of the emergency services department, was unable to access Mary's outpatient chart in the computer. While he could see that she had been an inpatient years before, none of her recent clinic records were available in the Electronic Medical Record forcing him to ask about her history, medications, and allergies. Her daughter, Joanna, had kept Mary's records on a home computer, but the CD she brought into the ER was unlabeled. Dr. Lobson did his best to explain why the

L. Einbinder et al. (eds.), *Transforming Health Care Through Information:*
Case Studies, Health Informatics, DOI 10.1007/978-1-4419-0269-6_9,
© Springer Science+Business Media, LLC 2010

hospital needed to be careful about accepting outside media, and set the CD aside. After quickly diagnosing Mary's pneumonia, Dr. Lobson admitted her to 3 West with a STAT order for intravenous D-Micen, a new antibiotic that he promised would rapidly improve her condition.

Up on the floor, a second "glitch" appeared. A communication problem delayed delivery of the drug request to the pharmacy. Jim Kane, a 3 West floor nurse on the second half of a double-shift, tried in vain to locate the medication in the unit's medication cabinet. After prompting from Mary's daughter and a heated conversation with the pharmacy, he finally received the medication and prepared the I.V. – but there were problems here too. After finding a dead battery on the wireless barcode scanner (required at Highland for all medication administration), the nurse used a backup device to successfully scan Mary's wristband and her badge. When he read the medication label, however, the computer sounded a loud warning beep. Emily knew now that the alert was justified – the outpatient clinic records showed an allergy to D-Micin class of drugs; the nurse, however, tired and overwhelmed, gave in to the family's pressure to "just read it with your eyes" and the computer alert went unheeded. Minutes later, Mary suffered a severe allergic reaction sending her into cardiac arrest.

After relating the chain of events to Steven, she leaned back and took off her reading glasses. "How can all this go wrong at the same time?" she asked.

Steven moved his mouse over a crowded screen full of program icons, snippets of programming code, and layered windows flashing green, yellow, and red stoplights. "All of our systems are connected." He explained, bringing a complex diagram of boxes, circles, and a myriad of arrows up on his computer screen. "Last Thursday night we were upgrading the software on our integration engine," he said, pointing to a circle near the center of the diagram, "and ran into some unexpected communication problems with different systems after we moved in the new code." "So this prevented Mary's outpatient medication and allergies from showing up in the ER?" asked Emily. "Yes, and it interrupted communications between our order entry systems in the ER and the pharmacy." "And the barcode devices on 3 West?" continued Emily. "Well, we've had problems with those keeping their charge after a full shift, but I'm glad the nurse thought to use the wired backup." "He did." Emily sighed, "Unfortunately, it alerted him to a drug allergy and he ignored it." "Oh, my. I'm told that this happens a lot because we've set the threshold for alerts so low and sometimes the labels don't print very clearly." "Wow." said Emily, shaking her head. "Did her outpatient allergy documentation catch up with her after she was admitted? It appears that this alert was legitimate and would have prevented her reaction." "Yes, I think so." Steven paused. "Was Mary OK after all this?" "They had to call a code, but she did just fine after discontinuing the D-Micen. It was a close call." The two sat in silence for a moment. Emily gathered her papers and stood up to leave. "Thank you, so much, Steven. Can I call you if I need any more information?"

Joanna's Story

Joanna couldn't quite believe what was happening. Highland Medical Center had an outstanding reputation for being both "high tech" and "high touch." Tonight, however, gremlins seemed to be conspiring against getting her mother, Mary, the help she needed so badly. After days of feeling weak and fighting off a bad cough, Mom could barely get a breath and was burning up with fever. Around midnight, Joanna and her father decided to get Mary to the emergency room. At first, Joanna felt good about the care they were getting. Dr. Kirk Lobson immediately diagnosed Mary with pneumonia, and moved quickly to have her admitted and started on antibiotics. But it was in the emergency department that things first started to go wrong. Despite being a Highland Clinic patient for years, the computer seemed to think that Mary hadn't been seen since she delivered Joanna, over twenty years before! To make matters worse, the CD she brought with Mom's personal health record couldn't be read on the hospital's machines. "Wasn't that the point of keeping computerized records," she wondered with irritation? The doctor tried to be reassuring, "We won't worry about the computer now," he said, though visibly annoyed. "Let's get you up to the floor. You'll feel better once we start you on the IV antibiotics." Things quickly went from bad to worse. After being moved to 3 West, Mary's breathing became even more of a struggle and the promised medicine was nowhere to be found. Joanna went to confront the nurse. She found him at the nurse's station punching buttons on what looked like an automated teller machine. He leaned heavily on the device, and judging from his appearance, he had already put in a long shift. "I'm so sorry," he said, "but, there's a problem with the pharmacy computers. I'll call down right away." "Damn right you will," she thought to herself before going back into her mother's room. A few minutes later, the nurse, looking even more haggard, appeared in the doorway of Mary's room wheeling an I.V. stand, a packet of tubing, and a large bag of clear liquid. "At last," Joanna said, not disguising her anger. The nurse rolled a stool close to Mary's bed and arranged his I.V. kit on top of the sheets. After tying a tourniquet around her arm and finding a vein, he looked up at Joanna and said "it won't be long now. She'll feel much better as soon as we get this going." He looked as though he could have used an I.V. himself as he swiveled around to face the bedside computer console. After logging on, he punched a few keys and produced a small barcode scanner from a plastic stand. Turning once again to the bed, he pointed the device at Mary's wrist bracelet and pulled the trigger. Nothing happened. He pulled the trigger again, and again, but there was no sound or laser flash. "What is it now?" insisted Joanna. "Um, I think the battery is dead." he said, not looking up to meet her glare. He brightened for a moment and said, "Don't worry though, I have a backup." Turning back to the side table, he produced a second device from a drawer, tethered to the computer by a thick cable. This time, there was a satisfying "beep" as he read the barcode on Mary's arm band. Joanna relaxed for a moment, but was startled seconds later to hear a loud "be-boop, be-boop, be-boop" coming from the scanner as he read the medication bag. The nurse froze, a look of confusion on his face. He read the bag again, and again came the dreadful warble. Frustration and anger welled up inside of Joanna. Her mother was getting worse by the minute, and now another stupid machine was preventing her from getting the medication she needed. "Read...It...With...Your...Eyes" she said slowly, her voice trembling.

Jim's Story

Jim was long past being ready to end a double shift. Tonight 3 West was shorthanded again, and he had agreed to stay over and handle an ER admit with pneumonia. In addition to managing twice his normal patient load, there were problems with the unit's medication cabinet, a nasty argument with the pharmacy ("I don't care what it says in YOUR computer..." he recalled saying), an anxious and upset family, and the final straw, two bedside scanners that were on the blink.

As he finished the last of his charting before finally going home he heard the scream from the hallway. "Someone please help my mother!"

It was the ER patient's daughter, and she was already angry about the delay in getting her mother's antibiotics started. He tried his best to keep his composure as she watched him struggle with the bedside medication scanners – first, a dead battery (the wireless units never seemed to last a full shift without needing to be recharged), and then, a scanning error on the I.V. bag label.

The barcodes from the pharmacy had been reading poorly with the scanners lately, and the thought of calling back down for a new label after his argument with the tech was just too much. Under the daughter's withering glare, he did what she asked and crosschecked the paperwork, the med sheet, and Mary's armband visually. Everything checked out. With the I.V. started, he had just returned to the nursing station to finish up and clock out.

The daughter was frantic. Jim stood up, knocking charts off the desk, and rushed into Mary's room where he found her looking even worse than when she had come to the floor – pale, sweating, and unresponsive. A thousand thoughts ran through his mind as he checked her vital signs. "I have a code in 314!" he yelled into the small communication device hanging from the lanyard around his neck, "I have a code in 314!"

Conclusion

We cannot help but feel sorry for the patient, her daughter Joanna, and poor Jim, the nurse. In this highly automated hospital, how could this series of serious "glitches" have been prevented?

Section III
Organizational Impact and Evaluation

Organizational Impact and Evaluation.............................. 103
  Cynthia S. Gadd

Chapter 10
The Implementation of Secure Messaging 107
  Zhou Yan

Chapter 11
Who Moved My Clinic? Donnelly University Pediatric
  Rehabilitation: The Wheelchair Clinic 115
  Fredrick Hilliard

Chapter 12
OncoOrders: The Early Years 127
  Chris Raggio and Judith W. Dexheimer

Chapter 13
Implementing a Computerized Triage System in the Emergency
  Department 135
  Scott R. Levin, Daniel J. France, and Dominik Aronsky

Chapter 14
Medication Barcode Scanning: Code "Moo": Dead COW................. 155
  Laurie L. Novak and Kathy S. Moss

Organizational Impact and Evaluation

CYNTHIA S. GADD

Organizational Impact and Evaluation[1]

The cases in this section focus on system development and implementation, and may be discussed in those contexts, of course. However, they also present an opportunity to pose the question of how general evaluation principles could be applied to study their often wide-ranging impacts within health care organizations. The following discussion contrasts traditional approaches to evaluation in biomedical informatics, which typically focus on the *what* questions, with sociotechnical and program evaluation approaches, and which provides more opportunities to explore the *how* and *why* questions that inform our understanding of organizational impacts.

The What

Evaluation methods in biomedical informatics must address a wide range of information resources, and an equally wide range of questions that can be asked about them, from technical characteristics to organizational issues. There are invariably many actors in health information technology (HIT) projects, including developers, users, and patients; all of whom may have different perspectives on what questions to ask and how to interpret the answers (some of which are changing over time). This complexity necessitates a wide array of empirical methods, including subjectivist designs that emphasize qualitative approaches, and a dynamic evaluation process. In contrast, research, including the logical-positivist/objectivist (or quantitative) traditions long dominant in biomedicine, serves the focused question or problem, excluding from a study as many extraneous variables as possible. It is not surprising that the overwhelming tendency in biomedical informatics evaluation over the past 25 years has been to prefer the use of the familiar study designs that emphasize quantitative approaches and methods, such as the Randomized Controlled Trial (RCT), even when they are not amenable to the questions to be answered.[1]

---

[1] Based on excerpts from Johnson KB, Gadd C, Playing smallball: approaches to evaluating pilot health information exchange systems. J Biomed Inform. 2007 Dec;40(6 Suppl):S21-S26, reprinted here with permission.

The How and Why

Stoop and Berg[2] point out that the dominance of RCTs has been questioned for years. In addition to general critiques, such as prejudice for an overly narrow definition of science, and the difficulty in separating the HIT intervention from its sociological entanglements, RCTs give "hard data" on a very constrained set of variables, leaving many more valuable questions of how and why, and under what circumstances unaddressed. They argue that managerially-focused evaluations should emphasize designs that focus on qualitative methods *integrated* with quantitative techniques that are less rigorous (and more widely applicable) than RCTs. They further suggest that in addition to using qualitative methods as "exploratory" steps or primarily for triangulation, the outputs of quantitative research, including "modest" before-after designs, can benefit from qualitative interpretation, e.g., to understand the consequences of downtime on performance of care.

The When

In addition to the philosophical grounds of evaluation, there is the issue of aligning evaluation questions, and methods with the developmental stages through which HIT typically progresses. Stead and colleagues[3] advised investigators to subdivide applied informatics research projects into steps, and tailor the evaluation to each step; the key idea is that a relationship exists between a developmental stage of a project and the level of evaluation that is appropriate. Five developmental stages are defined: Specification, Component development, Combination of components into a system, Integration of system into environment, Routine use; as well as five evaluation levels: Definition, Laboratory bench, Laboratory field, Remote field validity, Remote field efficacy. In their three stages of technology assessment, Fuchs and Garber[4] distinguish Stage 2 efficacy studies, which focus on process measures (e.g., degree of compliance with a reminder), from Stage 3 effectiveness studies, which directly evaluate health and economic outcomes (e.g., whether use of a cancer screening reminder lowered mortality).

In another approach to calibrating the type and timing of evaluation, Friedman uses an analogy from baseball to compare "powerball" evaluation, in which all evaluation resources are saved for an RCT of an extremely mature HIT project, to "smallball" evaluation, in which a succession of smaller, focused evaluation studies are conducted across the life-cycle of the project.[5] The value of smallball evaluation is seen in its potential for self-correction in the design and implementation of the project. Friedman argues that smallball evaluation studies can address needs that are of particular importance to community-based informatics interventions, such as health information exchanges: needs assessment, prototype testing, understanding usage (or lack of), and exploring the effects of the intervention when logistical or ethical constraints operating in community settings prevent randomization and blinding.

The What Revisited: Evaluation of "Messy" HIT

Berg[6] offers an approach drawn from sociotechnical science for understanding how the choice of HIT evaluation methods is necessarily grounded in recognition of the "messy" nature of healthcare practice as heterogeneous networks of people, tools, routines, etc. within specific socio-political contexts. This approach casts doubt on work as "rational" – represented in workflow diagrams and clinical pathways, but rather sees it as unfolding in the doing. Additionally, qualitative methods are deemed essential to study the network of changes resulting from HIT implementation, such as tasks, roles and responsibilities, and cultural notions of privacy and quality, as well as the fluidity of structural change inherent in healthcare organizations. Taken all together, these tumultuous interactions emphasize the simultaneous transformation of tool and practice.[7]

Another Why: Evaluation as "Useful Research"

Viewing HIT implementations from a sociotechnical perspective – as unfolding in heterogeneous networks of people, tools, roles, systems, processes and within specific socio-political contexts – allows us to generalize them as a type of social program (in which information technology is one component), and therefore amenable to the philosophies and techniques that are used in the field of *program evaluation* to determine if a program "works." Patton defines program evaluation as "the systemic collection of information about the activities, characteristics, and outcomes of programs to make judgments about the program, improve program effectiveness, and/or inform decisions about future programming." (Patton, 1996, p. 23) Program evaluation developed, particularly in the U.S., in the context of the Great Society programs of the 60s and 70s, including projects focused on education, health, housing, employment, urban renewal, welfare, and family programs. Extraordinary sums were invested, but the means of knowing what happened and why were not available. Early expectations for evaluation were focused on guiding funding decisions, separating successful programs from unsuccessful ones, and eventually grew to include helping improve programs as they were implemented.[8]

Professionalization of evaluation brought standards, foremost of which was that evaluation should be useful, i.e., evaluations should be judged by their utility and actual use. From these professional standards, evolved a distinction between evaluation research – undertaken to discover new knowledge, test theories, establish truth, and generalize across time and settings – and program evaluation – undertaken to inform decisions, identify improvements, and provide information about programs within contextual boundaries of time, place, values, and politics.[8] Cronbach and Suppes[9] described this as the difference between conclusion-oriented and decision-oriented inquiry.

The Who

Utilization-focused evaluation takes program evaluation one step further in that it is "done for and with specific, intended users for specific, intended uses."[8] This approach narrows the often large field of potential stakeholders who focus the evaluation to those who will use the evaluation data – the specific people who understand, and value evaluation should focus the evaluation: what questions will provide information that they care about and that will be relevant for their future action. Substantial research supports what Patton and others have identified the *personal factor* – the presence of an identifiable individual or group who personally care about the evaluation and the findings it generates (the "users") – as the single most important predictor of evaluation utilization. (Note that the "user" here is not necessarily the same as is typical in IT settings, i.e., the person who interacts with the IT system.)

Each of the cases that follow provides an opportunity to ask the questions necessary to understand the impacts of the HIT being designed and implemented:

- What impacts should be studied?
- How did these impacts happen?
- Why did these impacts happen?
- When should evaluation be done and how does timing affect the choice of methods used?
- Why and for whom do we do evaluation?
- How can we hope to evaluate impacts with the evolving, often messy nature of HIT?

References

1. Friedman CP, Wyatt J. *Evaluation methods in medical informatics.* 2nd ed. New York: Springer; 2006.
2. Stoop AP, Berg M. Integrating quantitative and qualitative methods in patient care information system evaluation: guidance for the organizational decision maker. *Methods Inf Med.*. 2003;42(4):458-462.
3. Stead WW, Haynes RB, Fuller S, et al. Designing medical informatics research and library-- resource projects to increase what is learned. *J Am Med Inform Assoc.*. 1994;1(1):28-33.
4. Fuchs VR, Garber AM. The new technology assessment. *N Engl J Med.*. 1990;323(10):673-677.
5. Friedman CP. "Smallball" evaluation: a prescription for studying community-based information interventions. *J Med Libr Assoc.*. 2005;93(4 Suppl.):S43-S48.
6. Berg M. Patient care information systems and health care work: a sociotechnical approach. *Int J Med Inform.*. 1999;55(2):87-101.
7. Berg M. *Rationalizing medical work: decision-support techniques and medical practices.* Cambridge, MA: MIT Press; 1997.
8. Patton MQ. *Utilization-focused evaluation.* 2nd ed. Beverly Hills: Sage Publications; 1986.
9. Coleman JS, Cronbach LJ, Suppes P. National Academy of Education. Committee on Educational Research *Research for tomorrow's schools: disciplined inquiry for education; report.* New York: Macmillan; 1969.

10
The Implementation of Secure Messaging

Zhou Yan

Like every other morning, Dave Foster poured himself a cup of coffee, walked to his study, turned on his computer, and started a new work day. Dave owns a home-based business which requires him to spend most of his work day in front of a computer.

Dave always begins each morning by checking his email. There were several emails waiting in the inbox on this particular morning. One of the emails immediately grabbed his attention. It was sent from the VUMC Patient Portal. He anxiously opened it. The email had only one paragraph: You have a new lab result. Please log in to Patient Portal to view the detail.

Dave had not been feeling very well recently. He had been experiencing inexplicable fatigue. The previous week, he went to see Dr. Fox, his primary physician. Dr. Fox ordered a radiology study and told him that the results should be available in a couple of days.

Dave logged in to the Patient Portal and found the lab results page. Sure enough, a new radiology report had been posted. Dave read the report carefully, almost word by word. Then at the bottom of the report, the words "possible thyroid cancer" jumped off the page. Dave felt as though his heartbeat suddenly stopped. After several minutes of shock, Dave clicked the "message your doctor" link and typed a message to Dr. Fox to ask for verification.

The time seemed to have stood still. It seemed forever before Dave received a reply from Dr. Fox, although it had only been an hour. Dr. Fox had read his report again and expressed that he felt very sorry he had missed the mention of possible cancer the first time he read the report.

An operation was quickly scheduled in the earliest available time slot. One week later, the operation had been successfully completed. Because thyroid cancer was diagnosed and treated at an early stage, no further threat was expected.

"Doctors are human, and human beings make mistakes," said Dr. Fox when he later discussed this story with other people. "I am so thrilled that the patient was able to catch the mistake and take action. I would say that this feature saved the patient's life." Dr. Fox is one of the doctors who had always been considered as computer savvy by his colleagues. He had been eagerly anticipating the secure messaging feature of the Patient Portal. He volunteered to be one of the first few doctors to participate in and use this new feature with all of his patients. Dave is one of the patients to whom Dr. Fox suggested trying the messaging feature in the Patient Portal.

L. Einbinder et al. (eds.), *Transforming Health Care Through Information: Case Studies*, Health Informatics, DOI 10.1007/978-1-4419-0269-6_10, © Springer Science+Business Media, LLC 2010

Background

In early 2001, Valley University Medical Center (VUMC), a leading research hospital in the southeastern United States, decided to create a Patient Portal web application to provide its patients with a secure web site to access their personal health records.

The initial plan was to purchase an existing web portal application and customize the software to meet the medical center's needs. After some marketing research, it was found that there were no existing web portals that could meet all of the medical center's requirements. The medical center then decided to develop its own Patient Portal. In the same year, a project team was formed and a software developer was hired to start the development.

The project team defined a set of features for the initial release. These features included enabling users to access their clinical and hospital bills, insurance information, and upcoming appointments.

The application was quickly developed and put into production within one year. The initial enrollment focused on VUMC employees. In spite of the project team's continuous effort to promote the site, enrollment remained low. The total number of users that signed up for an account was less than 3,000. There were approximately 500 logins per day.

In planning for the next version of Patient Portal, the project team decided to add more features. One of the planned features was to add a messaging capability to allow patients and doctors to communicate directly through email.

The timing was right for the secure messaging feature. Some doctors in the medical center had already begun communicating with their patients through regular internet emails, answering patient questions and processing prescription refill requests. At the same time, patient privacy concerns began attracting more public attention. The medical center was facing the challenge of meeting Health Insurance Portability and Accountability Act (HIPAA) regulations. Unsecured email sent between doctors and patients would definitely be a HIPAA violation.

The technical infrastructure for the secure messaging feature was already in place. VUMC had developed an in-house comprehensive electronic medical record system called SystemPanel. SystemPanel provides doctors and nurses with access to a patient's electronic medical record. It also has a built-in messaging feature to allow doctors and nurses to communicate with each other. Since the communication between patients and their clinicians is part of the patients' medical record which needs to be permanently recorded, it made perfect sense to build the new secure messaging feature on top of the SystemPanel application.

Project Planning Stage

The project team is led by Dr. J, the chief medical information officer of the medical center. Dr. J is a highly respected and a well-known physician in the medical center. He is the head of the primary adult care center and had just finished his MBA degree. People who are new to the team often wonder if the busy doctor has any personal time. The wonder continues when they learn that Dr. J is also a passionate bee keeper and Texas Hold'em poker player.

It does not take long for any team member to become familiar with Dr. J's work style. The meeting room is often filled with laughter from the jokes that Dr. J imposes on himself. If a team member poses a question to Dr. J by email, he should not be surprised to receive an answer from Dr. J within minutes, sometimes even a phone call.

Dr. J has been using the pilot release of the messaging feature to communicate with many of his patients. After several weeks of trial, the project team organized several user group meetings. Food was catered in after work and many patients came to the meeting despite the late hours of the day. The patients were varied in age groups and possessed different levels of computer skill. Most of the patients had been exchanging messages with Dr. J for several weeks.

Mrs. Wilson, a lady in her sixties, came with her husband. Mrs. Wilson has diabetes and has been seeing Dr. J for years. She couldn't stop talking about how easy it is for her to get her prescriptions refilled by simply sending a message. Mrs. Wilson's husband also came to the meeting. Mr. Wilson had been seeing a doctor in another local area hospital. After asking his doctor if they had something similar to the Patient Portal offered at the VUMC hospital, his doctor said that he had never even heard of such a thing. Mr. Wilson has since considered switching to a VUMC doctor.

Mr. Smith, another patient of Dr J's for years, is a computer professional who works for a local health insurance company. He loved the fact that he can ask questions about his symptoms at any hour of the day, even two o'clock in the morning. He said it is about time for the health industry to catch up with twenty-first century technology. Being an insider in the health insurance industry, Mr. Smith said he is concerned whether or not the other doctors at VUMC would use the new messaging feature, considering that this is an unpaid service provided by the doctors.

In addition to patients, members of the software development team were invited to attend the user group meeting. Jojo is one of the software developers who attended the meeting. Jojo is a software engineer who has been working on the Patient Portal development team for years. She has witnessed many changes in the Patient Portal application over the years. Her biggest frustration has been the luke-warm patient participation rate. This was her first opportunity to meet and talk to "real-life" patients.

After hearing the patients' positive feedback and hearing many requests for the messaging feature, Jojo felt renewed excitement. Jojo said, "It really felt great to be involved. As a developer, we often have our own way of thinking about what a user might want, but our ideas could be very different from what the user really wants. I hope we have more meetings like this."

User Interface Issues

The Patient Portal project team made the decision that the new portal messaging feature should leverage the existing SystemPanel messaging feature. This decision was made based on several factors. First, SystemPanel had gained a broad user base across VUMC clinics. Physicians and nurses were very familiar with the SystemPanel user interface. Second, after several years of operation, SystemPanel had proven its maturity and reliability in the institution.

The next step was to bring the Patient Portal development team and the SystemPanel development team together to nail down the technical details. The project teams very quickly found out that this was not a trivial task.

Although both teams belong to the VUMC, the two teams are managed by different departments. The two teams are physically located in two different buildings separated by a 15 min commute. The software developers in each team use different computer languages and frameworks. The development methodology that had been adopted by each team was dramatically different as well.

Several meetings were arranged between the two development teams to discuss technical details of building the secure messaging feature.

The first key decision was made quickly and unanimously. Each portal user will be given a message basket similar to the ones used by each physician. The SystemPanel team will be in charge of the creation and maintenance of these baskets.

The second key decision was much more involved. In order to decide how the new messaging feature should appear in the Patient Portal web page, the Patient Portal team proposed to maintain a look and feel consistent with the rest of the portal application. This would require the SystemPanel team to provide a set of application programming interfaces (APIs) to expose the internal SystemPanel functions as services. The SystemPanel team strongly resisted this proposal. One of the major reasons given was the lack of resources and time required to build and maintain the APIs.

After several meetings without reaching an agreement, the Patient Portal project team decided to give up the uniform user interface requirement and adopted a compromise solution. The Patient Portal would open a "window" inside its page which directly exposes the SystemPanel user interface. As a result, a Patient Portal user would see exactly the same user interface that the physicians and nurses would see.

This design approach resulted in many complaints from the portal users after the first launch. The SystemPanel user interface was designed very differently from that of a conventional email client. In order to fit into physician's busy work flow, the message baskets were presented as text only with no icons or graphics. Messages were displayed in a small font in order to fit as many messages as possible on one page. This user interface had worked well with physicians due to the compact interface design which required minimal navigation. The same user interface did not work well with the portal users who were accustomed to the user interface of more conventional email programs. Some of the specific complaints were:

- Users do not see the familiar icons used by popular email programs such as Outlook.
- Users report that the font looks different and difficult to read because it is so small.
- When users receive new messages, they do not know how to open it, because the subject line does not look like a hypertext link.
- Another frequent complain came from users who use web browsers other than the Microsoft Internet Explorer (IE) browser. Users who use the Patient Portal with Firefox and Safari web browsers often had problems opening the SystemPanel "window" inside the portal page.

The root of this problem is that the SystemPanel application was originally designed to be compatible only with the IE web browser. This design decision was made based on the VUMC IT infrastructure at that time. Physicians and nurses access SystemPanel application by using the clinical work stations (CWS) which are located throughout the hospital and clinical areas. The CWS computers are maintained by the VUMC IT department. All VUMC CWS computers run the Microsoft Windows operating system and the Microsoft IE web browser.

Policy Issue

An issue was quickly raised during one of the project meetings: how should unattended messages be handled?

The first challenge is how to handle unattended messages on the physician side.

"If someone uses the system to communicate an order to a nurse or patient's symptom to a doctor, and the message is not read by that doctor, serious harm could result. In addition, people will not use a system a second time if they find it to be unresponsive the first time. It is imperative that messages be answered reliably if the system is going to succeed," said the project chair, Dr. J.

The second challenge is equally important: How should the Patient Portal handle "unattended" messages on the patient side? What happens if the patient is not responding to messages sent by his physicians? What if the patient's email address has been changed and the patient fails to notify the physician's office?

The project team defined a set of policies to handle both challenges:

Policy 1: When a provider sends a message to a patient, the application will force the provider to specify a number of "bounce-back" days ranging from 1 to 14 days, based on the urgency of the message. When messages are not opened by a patient within the specified number of "bounce-back" days, the physician will automatically be notified and another means of communication, such as a telephone call, will be required to contact the patient.

Policy 2: A system audit report will be generated every Thursday morning. Except for messages explicitly put on hold, if no action (at least viewing the message) has been taken on a message within the past seven days, the message will be included in the audit report. The physician's office would thus be notified of the "unattended" message. The audit result is also sent to the clinic medical directors. Repeat offenders receive additional prodding.

These policies have proven effective. After two years of weekly audits, results have improved dramatically. In some recent weeks, unopened messages have dwindled to as few as one-fifth of 1%. More than 30,000 messages are sent each week, and in one recent week, only 66 were unattended, compared with more than 3,000 unattended messages per week before the audits began.

Security Issue

With HIPAA requirements in mind, the project team has placed significant emphasis on the security requirement of the messaging feature. It was decided early on that communication between the patient's browser and Patient Portal server will be encrypted.

Richard Foster, the Medical Center security officer, was invited to several of the design meetings. Richard had requested that all passwords must be at least eight characters long and can be any combination of letters and numbers and must contain at least one number, one upper case letter and one lower case letter.

This strict password policy was intended to protect users' sensitive data from being compromised, but at the same time, it has also presented difficulties for authorized users to remember their passwords. During the initial launch of the Patient Portal application, the Medical Center help desk received a significant volume of phone calls from patients reporting Patient Portal login problems. The majority of these calls were from users who had forgotten or mistyped their passwords. This problem was relieved to some degree by the addition of a function which allows users to reset their passwords by answering a series of secret questions with answers known only by the user.

Rolling Out to Clinics

In October 2005, after several months of intense development and testing, a new version of the Patient Portal application was ready for release. One of the major changes in this version was a new portal page called "Messaging Your Doctor's Office." This page can be accessed by all portal users with full access rights.

After logging into the portal web site, the user will see all new messages, as well as previous ones. Unread messages are highlighted to draw the user's attention to messages that have not been opened. Replying to a message requires only a single click. Starting a new message is as simple as selecting a doctor's name from a list of VUMC doctors that the patient has previously seen.

Also included with the new release is a separate Patient Portal Administration Application (PPAA). The PPAA is designed for use by authorized medical center staff to manage portal users' accounts. An authorized clinical staff member can create a new account, delete an existing account, resolve duplicate medical record numbers, and most importantly, upgrade a user's access level in order to use the secure messaging feature.

Cindy Clark and her team were ready and eager to roll out the new version to all clinics in the Medical Center. It was decided early on that the roll out would be conducted in a staged manner. The team would focus on one clinic at a time. Cindy and her team would personally visit the clinic to help to set up the application and answer any questions.

Clinic1 was the first clinic on the list. This clinic is located in the Green Hills area and sees a fairly large number of patients each day. Beth Thomson, a nurse practitioner, met with Cindy on a Monday morning at the scheduled roll out date.

"This is simple, let me show you how this works," said Cindy Clark as she helped Beth open a new IE browser window and navigate to the web address of the PPAA site. "Just log in with your VUMC id and password here and click the..." Before Cindy could finish the sentence, Beth interrupted, "I am afraid this won't work," Cindy looked up from her computer with a noticeable frown and a puzzled look on her face. "Why not?" she asked.

Beth sighed, "We are so swamped with patient visits every day, and on top of that, we have all these administrative tasks to complete. We just don't have the time to bring up another application and type in yet another username and password." After a short pause, Beth said again, "You can ask other nurses around here, I am sure they would say the same thing."

Conversations with other people in the clinic confirmed Beth's prediction. Feeling frustrated, Cindy walked around the clinic floor. She noticed that several nurses were working in front of clinical workstations (CWS); all of them were busy entering data into SystemPanel with fluency.

Cindy immediately came back to Beth. "How about we add a PPAA link inside SystemPanel? You wouldn't need to bring up another browser and remember the web address to PPAA!" Cindy offered and eagerly looked at Beth's face. "That might work," said Beth as she considered the possibility. "And there is more," Cindy continued. "If you are logged into SystemPanel, you wouldn't need to log in to the PPAA again, because the same login works for both applications." said Cindy. Beth smiled and said, "Now you are talking!"

Cindy came back to develop the team and requested that they make the changes. The developers responded, "It's just couple of simple clicks, why is it such a big deal?" The developers had a hard time understanding the change request. Cindy managed to convince the developers that it is critical to get the nurses' buy in. "Without their support, we can't roll out to any clinic." said Cindy.

During the following month, Cindy and her team continued to roll out the application to all of the clinics on campus. She then moved on to off-campus clinics, and even to several that are located outside of Tennessee.

From June 2007 through October 2007, the Patient Portal gained 426 new registrants per week, the total number growing from 28,188 users to 37,145 in just 5 months.

Each day, between 1,500 and 2,000 patients visit the Patient Portal. The number of new user sign-ups up to the site continues to amaze the development team. The system log showed that majority of administrative tasks was conducted from the links embedded in the SystemPanel application. Cindy was right after all.

Conclusion

The release of the secure messaging feature, together with other features added in the new version of the Patient Portal has increased the overall usage of the site. Comparing to the version before the secure messaging feature was added; the total number of users signed up has increased from about 2,500 to over 37,000. The daily login has increased from 300 to over 2,000.

The various policies applied to the secure messaging feature have proved to be effective. Unattended messages rate has dropped from 15% to the recent 0.2% within two years.

The integration architecture between the Patient Portal and SystemPanel has ensured a quick implementation. However, the inherited technical difficulties have resulted in problems requiring further design of the user interface, usability, and security.

The clinic managers had mostly positive feedback regarding the messaging feature and the Patient Portal application. The common benefits witnessed by the clinic managers include:

- Ability to get result quickly to patients,
- Reduced the work load for clinical staff.

The physicians' responses regarding the messaging feature are mixed. On the basis of a limited number of survey results, most of the responses are positive due to several factors:

- Improve the quality of patient care by involving patient in their own treatment.
- Able to deliver test results more quickly and easily.
- Help with the daily work flow, allowing patients' questions to be answered at a convenient time.

There were few negative responses regarding the fear of law suits, extra work load, and unpaid service.

Some doctors are sheltered from the messaging feature. Their main interactions with the patients are in person. The messages are handled by clinic nurses and administrative assistants.

Questions

1. How would you evaluate the rollout of the Patient Portal?
2. What groups would you include in your evaluation process?
3. What quantitative and qualitative measures would you include?

References

Ward, Getahn. The Tennessean Business Section: E-medicine: It has strong devotees but privacy issues slow growth of valuable programs. http://www.tennessean.com/apps/pbcs.dll/article?AID=/20080316/BUSINESS01/803160386/1003/NEWS01; 2008 Accessed 16 03 08.

Govern, Paul. The Reporter: Convenience drives My Health growth. http://www.mc.VUMC.edu/reporter/index.html?ID=6015; 2007 Accessed 30 11 07

11
Who Moved My Clinic? Donnelly University Pediatric Rehabilitation: The Wheelchair Clinic

FREDRICK HILLIARD

Introduction to Children's Hospital Pediatric Rehabilitation

Background

The Department of Pediatric Rehabilitation Services at Donnelly University is a subsidiary of the Children's Hospital at this healthcare institution. The Department of Pediatric Rehabilitation Services is used by many people around the state. Many families travel several hours to receive the quality service that this department has to offer. On a daily basis the department serves approximately 100 patients. During the course of one year there are approximately 25,000 visits to the clinic. Therapists were not limited to visiting patients in a clinical setting. In addition, they would travel to specialized schools to facilitate treatment in the school setting.

Mission and Goals

This department's goal is to improve motor control and provide assistive technology services to children who suffer from impairments, functional limitations, disabilities, or changes in physical function and health status resulting from injury, disease or other causes. For example, therapies are provided to children with fractures, sprains, head injury, spinal cord injuries, congenital abnormalities, sensory processing disabilities, learning disabilities and neuro-developmental impairments.

In conjunction with treating their wide variety of patients, the department endeavors to integrate the family and caregivers of the child into the child's rehabilitation in order to maximize success. The family and caregivers will be involved in developing the child's treatment plan, and parent training will be provided to ensure proper implementation of home programs.

Available Resources and Services Provided

The staff of the Pediatric Rehabilitation department is composed of individuals with various specialties. Primarily, there are three types of therapists in this department: Physical Therapists (PT), Occupational Therapists (OT) and Speech Therapists (Speech-language Pathologist).

L. Einbinder et al. (eds.), *Transforming Health Care Through Information:*
Case Studies, Health Informatics, DOI 10.1007/978-1-4419-0269-6_11,
© Springer Science+Business Media, LLC 2010

PT focus on improving and maximizing a child's mobility. They are trained to observe and evaluate a child's functional mobility, assess the primary areas that can be improved and implement the best methods of treatment. Their treatment is designed to promote physical abilities, fitness and wellness. PT may recommend splinting and casting, bracing/orthotics, wheelchair and seating, and adaptive equipment, in cases where they believe these technologies will improve the long-term quality of life of the patient.

OT are concerned with observing and evaluating how children perform in everyday contexts. Treatments focus on helping patients regain or develop skills necessary which will be used in the child's everyday life. For children, this means developing life skills and tasks that will enable them to engage in their environment as independently as possible through exercises and task-related activities. Often in order to fully engage younger children these activities will be disguised as play. Formatting the therapy in this manner also, encourages the children and their families to engage in the treatments at home.

One area where physical therapy and occupational therapy techniques are synergistically used to improve the quality of life of special patients is the Katie Darnell Wheelchair Clinic. The remainder of this case study will focus on the wheelchair clinic, its personnel, their interactions, the technology that is used in the clinic, and the effect that moving to a new location has on all of the clinic's stakeholders.

The Katie Darnell Wheelchair Clinic

Introduction

The wheelchair clinic is a part of the pediatric rehabilitation department which focuses on providing mobility solutions for patients ranging in age from toddlers to teenagers. The personnel of the wheelchair clinic supply products and services to patient's suffering from physical, sensory, cognitive or mental impairments all of which could result from a genetic disorder, disease, or injury. The clinic ensures that all treatments that are implemented fit each patient's biomechanical and motor control abilities. These characteristics are very important when deciding which type of chair is appropriate. For example, an adolescent patient with full cognitive ability and adequate motor-visual coordination but lacking the biomechanical ability to reach and manually push a wheelchair would be an ideal candidate for a power chair. Two other types of wheelchairs are both mechanically powered, one type is pushed by the patient and the other type is pushed by another individual.

Background

The wheelchair clinic is open twice a week for four hours a day. At the time of this case study the clinic was open on Monday from 8 a.m.–12 p.m. and on Thursday from 1–5 p.m. Although, these times are the "normal" office hours for the clinic, it is not uncommon for the therapists to stay at least an hour after the designated time. The information presented about the clinic is derived primarily from observations of clinic appointments that took place on Thursday afternoons.

The team of medical and technology professionals working in the clinic possessed a variety of backgrounds and expertise. The clinic personnel included two therapists, an occupational and a physical therapist, a vendor representative and a technician. Each therapist saw one patient every hour, so there were typically two appointments scheduled every hour. In spite of their differences in training, the two therapists of the wheelchair clinic provide the same services to their patients. For all appointments, each therapist was accompanied by one vendor representative and for appointments that required wheelchair adjustments or fittings a technician would accompany the vendor representative. Table 11.1 displays the personnel who contribute to the clinic's operation.

The patients seen in this wheelchair clinic were all under the age of 18. After a patient is older than 18 years old he or she must begin using the adult wheelchair clinic which is a part of the rehabilitation services in another part of the hospital. The wheelchair clinic is located at one of the most prominent health centers in the state. Therefore, the clinic receives many referrals from rural areas of the state where they do not have local clinics available. There were some patients who also came from neighboring states (four to six hour drive) to visit the clinic. The majority of these patients are from a lower socioeconomic status and have limited insurance which often makes it difficult for the therapist and vendor representative to provide the appropriate resources to the patient and their family.

Wheelchair Ordering Process

The process of acquiring a wheelchair is an arduous journey that involves several different people and groups over a significant period of time. The first step is that the patient's physician must write a prescription for a new wheelchair or other technology due to various health factors. The physician provides a copy of the prescription to the patient and often the physician will recommend the wheelchair clinic for the patient to fill the prescription.

At the wheelchair clinic the first step the patient undergoes is the preliminary evaluation. During the preliminary evaluation there are several steps of questioning and analysis which allow the therapist and vendor representative to determine the appropriate chair to meet the needs of the patient. Some of the steps that occur are acquisition of the patient's dimensions (height, thigh width, shoulder width, weight, length of upper and lower legs, etc.), and determining the patient's capabilities (motor control, visual acuity, etc.). The therapist also examines the patient physically by looking for marks or bruises on the patient's back due to lack of padding and determining flexibility of the patient's legs. In addition to assessing the patient, it is important to include the parents or primary caregiver(s) in this process to determine what features of the chair are necessities for the patient's everyday life. For example, aspects of the patient's everyday life that must be considered are: if the patient attends home school, public or private school; if the patient uses the school bus; if the parent must transfer patient out of chair, or can the patient transfer him or her self out of the chair.

The majority of the information collected is recorded into a computer by the therapist. However, some of this information is also pertinent to the vendor representative's records. Hence, the therapist and the vendor representative often work together during the measurement and recording process, where one will measure and the other will record the information. At the end of the evaluation appointment, the vendor representative and the therapist determine the best option for the patient and outline the required padding for the chair, measurements (size, seat depth, foot plate height, side

TABLE 11.1. Responsibilities of Wheel Chair Clinic Personnel and Referring Physicians

	Therapist	Vendor representative	Technician	Physician
Primary responsibility	Assess patients needs Determine requirements for wheelchair Inform parents and patient concerning proper use of chair Write LMN	Determine which chair is best for therapist's requirements and patient's age and size. Liaison between manufacturer and therapist Provide information to insurance company	Perform repairs, modifications and programming needs on chair	Write prescription for chair and other technologies the patient may need Primary source of care for the patient Source of information for parents
Required appointment attendance	All patient appointments in wheelchair clinic	All patient appointments in Wheelchair clinic	Appt. when chair is delivered to patient	None
Patient interaction	Primary contact for patient in wheelchair Clinic	Some patient interaction, when accessing wheelchair fit	Very little patient interaction	Primary point of contact for parents regarding patients overall health and needs
Follow-up requirements	Provides follow-up in the Wheelchair Clinic	Follow-up when necessary May make house calls	Follow-up when necessary May make house calls	Constant follow-up with patient

brace and head rest positioning, etc.). Information about the wheelchair is then presented parent/care giver, whom has the option of accepting that option or asking for another solution. The therapist and vendor representative often know which is best for the patient and have enough background and knowledge in the field to convince the parent if there are any reservations about the suggested wheelchair. The major concern for many parents about ordering the wheelchair is the expense that they will have to incur for what insurance does not cover. Fortunately, the vendor representative's expertise in dealing with insurance companies in this area often resolves many of these concerns.

After the parent consents to the order, the therapist uses a computer program to generate the Letter of Medical Necessity (LMN). The LMN details the needs and outlines the therapist's and vendor representative's rationale for choosing a particular wheelchair for the patient. The computer program generates a template for the LMN which reduces the therapist's time on the computer and increases the approval rate of the LMN. In addition to including information about the wheelchair, if the therapist determines there are other needs for the patient (i.e., a bath chair), these may also be included in the LMN. After composing the LMN, the vendor representative submits the letter to the physician for approval. This step ensures that the physician's intended treatment for the patient is being fulfilled. If the physician approves the LMN, it is then submitted to the patient's insurance company to request funding for the chair.

Acquiring approval from the insurance company is often the sticking point in this entire process. Some insurance companies take months to reply to the LMN from the vendor representative and if the reply is denied then the LMN must be revised with the hope of acquiring approval on the next submission. Many insurance companies will deny a request for a high end wheelchair if adequate justification is not presented in the LMN. This potential road block demonstrates the essential need for the therapist and vendor representative to present the best argument for their solution in the LMN.

The insurance company's approval allows the technology vendor representative to submit the work order with the technical and aesthetic information about the chair to the wheelchair manufacturer. There are many wheelchair manufacturers and the vendor representative is familiar with the types of chairs that exist and the best manufacturer for producing that specific wheelchair. Once the manufacturing process is complete the chair is delivered to the vendor representative. At the vendor representative's warehouse, the technician makes additional adjustments, if necessary, and the vendor representative along with the technician deliver the chair to the client at their next wheelchair clinic appointment.

The time between the initial evaluation and delivery of the wheelchair can range from two to six months. During this period of time it is possible that the patient has grown, gained weight or undergone other changes which may result in the patient fitting differently in the chair than that which was originally observed in the evaluation appointment. These changes typically do not result in the need to re-order the wheelchair, instead the therapist and vendor representative will put the patient in the wheelchair and instruct the technician to make mechanical adjustments that will customize the chair to the patient. Once the chair has been customized, the vendor representative and therapist will teach the parent how to use the chair (i.e., engaging brakes, folding the chair, disassembly/reassembly, etc.). Further, if the chair is manually propelled by the patient or is controlled by a joystick that the patient uses to direct movement, the patient must also be taught how to correctly maneuver the chair.

Patients of the Wheelchair Clinic

Integral to the effective function of the wheelchair clinic are the therapist, vendor representative and technician. However, none of these entities would exist if it were not for the needs of the patient. The Pediatric Rehabilitation Department makes an effort to always maintain the needs of the patient as a top priority. Keeping this in mind, the wheelchair clinic is highly dependent on defining the individual requirements for each patient. The following examples demonstrate the high variability and specificity that must be provided to every individual.

Billy is a 10 year old male suffering from muscular dystrophy. He and his family (mother, father and older brother) have been coping with this illness since his birth. The first wheelchair that was issued to Billy was a stroller chair, which required another person to push the chair. At his evaluation appointment the therapist determined that the overall muscular development of his arms, his visual-motor coordination and cognitive development were adequate for using a power chair. The power chairs grant the patient a great deal of independence, the model that was chosen had additional controls for lift, descent, and tilt. The descent feature was especially important to Billy's parents, because in his class the teacher does "story time" where the class sits on the floor in a circle. Billy's previous chair kept him at a height much greater than that of his peers during this time. However, this new feature allows him to lower his seat on the same level during "story time." This chair also had programing which allowed Billy's parents and teachers to set the speed of the power chair so that Billy did not hurt himself or others by driving the chair at top speed. The chair was customized to fit Billy and the control was turned inward to give him optimal control. Turning the controls inward also required reprograming, which was done by the vendor representative who connected the controls to her laptop and used a computer program to calibrate the controls. After the customization process was complete, Billy was taught how to drive the chair and make various types of turns.

Michelle is a 9-year old female who suffers from a neuroblastoma which has resulted in her reliance on a wheelchair. In spite of her illness Michelle is very high functioning with an adventurous and determined personality to accompany her abilities. She came in to her evaluation appointment in a chair that was almost falling apart. The area of the state she lives consists of many dirt roads and rocky areas that over time had a significant effect on the state of her first wheelchair. During her evaluation appointment the vendor representative made some adjustments to her current chair to account for the rugged terrain. The terrain issue makes Michelle an poor candidate for a power chair; instead she would be a better candidate for a manually powered chair with a sport design that is more suitable to her environment and her high level of functionality. This lightweight durable chair is best for Michelle and her family.

The two cases described above demonstrate the significant variability and detail that goes into choosing a wheelchair for a patient.

The effectiveness of the wheelchair clinic is reliant on several factors which change depending on the personnel, technology and space available. All of these factors were altered during observations of the wheelchair clinic, due to the clinic's move to a new location. These variables had a noticeable affect on the quality of care provided by the clinic, and the details of the changes are discussed below.

Change in Location

The Children's Hospital recently purchased a large, former retail space, and desig-nated certain departments to move there. Pediatric Rehabilitation Services was the first department to move to this new location.

The department's previous location had several small rooms, and the room that was allocated for the wheelchair clinic may have been one of the smallest. The room did not have adequate seating for families, primarily because of space limitations. In addi-tion, the therapists did not have any method of providing privacy to patients. In cases where patients brought family members it was sometimes necessary to lock the door because the patient and therapist would be working in the direct path of the door and if someone opened the door to quickly it may have injured the patient or clinic person-nel. The small space also limited the area where patients could test their new wheel-chairs and learn navigation techniques. For example, when Billy was learning to use his new power chair, he had to learn how to navigate the chair in the narrow hallway that was adjacent to the room. This limited his privacy and also required that the vendor representative and therapist leave the clinic while Billy was testing his new wheelchair. The final issue pertains to the layout of the clinic. The vendor represent-ative and therapists often needed to store various types of headrests, pads, sample wheelchairs and tools in a storage closet which was located outside of the room where the patients were located. If anything was ever needed from this room, the therapist, vendor repre-sentative or technician would have to leave the patient go to the store room, and come back after the item was retrieved. This arrangement took one of the team members away from the patient for a period of time.

The new location addressed several of the issues that were noticed with the old location. The size of the room used for the clinic was twice as large as the old location. The new space was large enough that patients testing wheelchairs are able to begin in the room and move out to the hallway if they choose. The new location had built in seating along the walls for the patient's families; it also had two therapy tables with overhead cur-tains that could be used to provide various private areas in the room. Another impor-tant change with the new location is that the room had a large supply closet connected to the wheelchair clinic. This feature allows the personnel to obtain supplies, parts and tools without having to leave the clinic room. Overall, the new location promotes more patient privacy, improves the quality of the treatment and allows the personnel to spend more time with the patient during the appointment.

This new location provides great benefits in terms of space and overall layout. However, there are some disadvantages to the new space. The first is related to the actual process of changing locations. Patients of the wheelchair clinic have approxi-mately two or three appointments, which may occur over a span of six months. Thus, one month after the move to the new location, patients were still going to the old loca-tion unaware of the wheelchair clinic's move to another place. This would cause patients to miss appointments and disturb the start times of appointments. This issue will most likely be resolved over time when patients begin to recognize the new loca-tion as the only location for the wheelchair clinic.

A second issue is related to staff members having to commute from the primary hospital to the new location. For example, one of the therapists who works in the wheelchair clinic also holds a managerial position in Pediatric Rehabilitation Services, which requires her to work in the primary hospital at times when she is not in the wheelchair clinic. Having to make this commute may become problematic if there are scheduling conflicts with her job at the primary hospital that could make her late for or unable to make appointments at the clinic. The other therapist works as a per diem employee and only comes in for the wheelchair clinic; therefore, scheduling and travel are not as much of an issue.

Technology Available

The information technology available to the therapists in the new location is much different than what was used in the old location. In the old location the therapists were anchored to a desktop station which was located in a way that required the therapist to turn their back to the patient when using the computer. This situation often made it difficult for the therapist to maintain eye contact with the patient and the family.

Approximately three months prior to moving to the new location, the wheelchair clinic implemented a new software program that would be used for developing the LMN, recording patient information and updating patient records. The new program is able to interface and transfer information, from the wheelchair clinic, to the programs used in the primary hospital. An issue that arose with the new program in the old location is that the per diem therapist was not formally trained on using the program. Instead, the full-time therapist was formally trained and was responsible for assisting the other therapist in learning the program and using it during appointments.

The new location implemented a few changes that would address the issue of the therapist being anchored to the desktop and not being able to move around the room with the patient. The new location did not have desktop computers in the wheelchair clinic. Instead, Pediatric Rehabilitation Services instituted a laptop program. They also placed furniture in the room which was more conducive to using the laptops. The therapists used light-weight rolling stools that allowed them to sit anywhere in the room. Instead of using desks, they used small rolling tables that were the perfect size for supporting a laptop. The therapists were also able to elevate and lower the table to suit their needs if they are sitting or standing. They installed wireless technology that was connected through a server to the main network at the primary hospital. These measures were implemented to grant the therapist more flexibility, increase the time spent with patients and increase the quality of care that patients receive.

The implementation of new technology at the clinic had several immediate benefits; however, there were some negative aspects, as well. First, the laptop program required the per diem therapist to come in twenty minutes earlier than normal because she would have to check-out a laptop and set up her work area. After completing her appointments she would then have to shut down and return the laptop. She regarded this as inconvenient and unnecessary. In addition, the rolling carts are an improvement on the immobile desktops; however, the rolling desks are still limited in the distance they can travel. The laptops must be plugged in the wall outlet which limits the distance it is able to travel. Further, if a therapist uses the elevation feature of the desk then the distance she can travel with the laptop is reduced. A few solutions, to this problem would be to use rolling carts with batteries that would act as a power source for the laptop, or to instruct the therapist to use the laptop's battery when they need to travel distances with the computer. Laptops are very different from desktops. For example, a person must understand how to use a touch pad instead of using an external mouse. The department did not provide any training for the therapists on how to appropriately use a laptop at the new location. Finally, the rolling stools that the therapists use lack the ergonomic support that a person using a computer would require. Although, this may seem like a small negative aspect, it is a very important feature that must be addressed. The therapist is often lifting patients or their chair, bending over the patient to do the examination and walking around with the patient during testing of the chair. All of these activities put stress on the therapists back and legs. Using furniture which lacks ergonomic support will decrease the quality of care that a therapist is able to provide, due to the development of lower back pain or pain in the legs or feet. These pains will cause the therapist to become distracted from the patient because more attention will be focused on their own discomfort.

Amenities Provided

The old location provided one unique amenity that was ideal for the wheelchair clinic. All families and patients were able to use valet parking which was located approximately thirty feet away from the check-in desk for the wheelchair clinic. This amenity was not only convenient for the patient and their family but it relieved a potential sticking point in the wheelchair clinic's process flow. The parking lots at the old location were a significant distance away from the primary hospital. Instead of the patient and their family having to walk a long distance or use a shuttle, they could be dropped off in front of the clinic's entrance. The valet parking amenity reduced the chances that a patient would be late due to attempting to find a parking space. The drop off area was also covered by an awning which is essential in times of inclement weather.

Currently, the new location does not have the amenity of valet parking. However, the parking lot at this location is directly in front of the entrance to the rehabilitation services office. Although, the need for valet parking is less at the new location, the need still exists. It would very difficult for a single patient or caregiver to push a wheelchair and hold an umbrella if it were raining. The farthest parking spaces from the front door are a significant walking distance away from the door. The other issue is that there is not an awning covering the door entrance. This means that in the even of inclement weather it is impossible to keep the patient or chair completely dry during the process of moving the patient to the car.

Team Communication

Vendor Representative-Therapist Relationship

The synergy of these two people contributes greatly to the patient's overall experience and the quality of care they will receive, during their two to three visits to the clinic. Therefore, it is important that these two individuals are comfortable with each other and understand their roles in providing patient care.

The old clinic's location size allowed the therapist and vendor representative to always be in close proximity to each other. The lack of distance between the two individuals promoted constant communication and collaboration. The old location did not appear to have any negative consequences on the relationship between the vendor representative and the therapist. However, one cost of the small space is that the vendor representative and therapist had very little privacy to discuss specific options for a patient, if it was ever desired. The result was that every conversation or idea that was discussed was also overheard by the patient and his or her family.

Therapist-Therapist Relationship

The relationship between the two therapists in the clinic, does not directly affect the quality of care for the patients in most cases. In some cases the therapists may collaborate regarding the patient's needs for a wheelchair. This is typically a rare occurrence because both therapists have patients during the normal clinic hours. Primarily, this relationship has been essential for the use of technology in the clinic.

While still in the old location the per diem therapist would have to ask the full-time therapist for assistance with using the new documentation software. The per diem therapist's lack of formal training with the software made the full-time therapist almost essential to the clinic. In one instance, the full-time therapist was unable to be in the wheelchair clinic, and the per diem therapist had technical problems with the software and tried for several minutes to resolve the issue herself. However, when she was not able to resolve the issue she had to leave the clinic and find another full-time rehabilitation employee that had received software training to resolve the problem.

There were also some technical difficulties at the new location. While at the new location there was a failure with the server connecting the per diem therapist's laptop to the primary hospital's network. This is a critical problem because the documentation software would not work properly unless the computer was connected to the network. In addition, the therapists use the computer to access patient records, which means that for a period of time the therapist did not have access to her patient's records. At the time the failure occurred both therapists were with a patient. The full-time therapist was beginning her assessment and did not need her computer immediately, however, the per diem therapist needed to begin constructing the LMN for a patient. The full-time therapist's computer was still working so they decided to quickly switch computers. While the vendor representative was working with the full-time therapist's patient, she called technical support to address the issue of the malfunctioning connection. This effectively distracted both therapists from attending to their patients, and increased the patients' time in the clinic. Both of these factors can have a negative impact on the patients' quality of care.

The Therapist-Therapist relationship is very important to maintaining the standard flow of clinic operations regarding the technology that is used in the clinic. The requirement for this relationship to exist remained the same in the old and new locations. The size of the room, amenities available or other effects does not diminish the necessity for this dynamic to exist. The relationship became even more essential with the transition from desktops that are hardwired to the network to laptops that are connected to the primary hospital through a remote wireless connection.

Conclusion

The wheelchair clinic is imperative to maintaining and improving the quality of life for all of its patients. The clinic is composed of several team members (therapists, technology vendor representatives, and technicians) that are essential to the success of the clinic. Each team member has specific roles that must be fulfilled in order for the patient's quality of care to be met. Recently, the clinic changed locations that caused alterations in the clinic's available space, technology, amenities and working relationships (i.e., therapist-vendor representative and therapist-therapist). The change did not seem to have a significant effect that would result in a dramatic decrease in the quality of care. Overall, the move to the new location has positively impacted the wheelchair clinic staff's ability to provide service and support for their patients. After addressing some of the disadvantages of the new location, clinic personnel will be able to provide optimal quality of care with adequate facilities and technological resources.

Questions

1. Pediatric Rehabilitation Service managers implemented a new software program less than three months before the move to the new location. This provided the therapists in the wheelchair clinic less than ten days to use the software in a clinical setting before the move to the new location. Technical dilemmas with the new software occurred in the old and new clinic. What do you believe are the primary repercussions from the technological malfunctions that were experienced in the new clinic?
2. The managers of the wheelchair clinic implemented the new documentation software at the old clinic. However, there were still integration difficulties at the new clinic. What other strategies do you believe the managers could have used to avoid this situation?
3. The wheelchair clinic functions based on three relationships (vendor-therapist, therapist-therapist and vendor-technician). Which relationship do you believe is most essential to the wheelchair clinic? Also, what measures can the managers of the clinic and clinic personnel take to ensure maximum efficiency of this relationship?
4. The primary sticking point of the wheelchair ordering process was discussed in this case. What changes in the process can be implemented to reduce the lag created by this sticking point?

References

Lorenzi NM, Riley RT. *Managing Technological Change: Organizational Aspects of Health Informatics*. 2nd ed. New York: Springer; 2003.

12
OncoOrders: The Early Years

Chris Raggio and Judith W. Dexheimer

Introduction to OncoOrders

This case study describes the development of an order-entry system in a chemotherapy clinic at Southwest Regional Medical Center. The system functions as a "whiteboard" and an organizational system for the Cancer Clinic. All of the systems were developed in-house at Southwest Regional by the Informatics Department. OrderAssistant, the order-entry system at Southwest Regional Hospital, has been in use in the wards for 7 years and has been a resounding success. A homegrown application, it was developed as an effort to supplant the cumbersome InVision system, which served previously as the computerized order-entry system at Southwest Regional. Although OrderAssistant is used in the inpatient environment, the designers felt that it could also be adapted to meet the Cancer Clinic outpatient's needs such as tagging orders with DRG/ICD-9 codes and delivering orders to a patient who may or may not be located in a bed. Late in the course of the OncoOrders project, it was realized that the orchestration of activity that occurred after patients checked in resembled the activity in the Emergency Department (ED). In both environments, patients were triaged, checked in, and had labs, tests, and clinic visits scheduled according to their needs. The electronic whiteboard employed in the emergency room has been largely successful and has greatly increased the efficiency of workflow. Aiming to capitalize on that success, the Steering Committee decided to enlist help from the ED whiteboard team to produce a whiteboard for the infusion room in the chemotherapy clinic. This new whiteboard would provide an at-a-glance display of where each patient was and what treatment they were undergoing. It would also give the nurses relief from having to track patients via paper logs and retrieve each lab result via the electronic medical record. All of this information could be viewed on the whiteboard. Having decided upon what a digital Cancer Clinic would look like, the challenge remained to adapt these two tools for use in an outpatient clinic comprising patient visit, lab work, and chemotherapy infusion.

Background

Southwest Regional Medical Center is an important medical center in the southwestern United States. This Cancer Clinic is the only comprehensive outpatient cancer clinic in the state. The clinic screens 120 patients per day including lab draws, clinic visits, and

L. Einbinder et al. (eds.), *Transforming Health Care Through Information: Case Studies*, Health Informatics, DOI 10.1007/978-1-4419-0269-6_12, © Springer Science+Business Media, LLC 2010

chemotherapy infusion. The patients may also receive adjuvant medications, consult other providers for comorbid health problems, undergo x-ray and CT imaging, and receive radiation therapy. The clinic is currently using a paper-based system to track and treat patients. The entire system is extremely reliant on a highly competent charge nurse to coordinate clinical care.

In 1998, the Cancer Clinic requested the Informatics Department if they could create an order-entry and patient tracking system to improve the quality of care for patients receiving chemotherapy. This system, when implemented, would help reduce the number of medication errors and the work-load on the charge nurse. The system would contain an order-entry system with rule sets to check for drug interactions and contraindications for a patient receiving chemotherapy.

Going beyond order-entry it would also allow the provider to create, in the abstract, the complete plan of care for the patient. This care plan would be robust and flexible – adapting to changing circumstances such as a missed appointment or adverse reaction to medication. As a stopgap solution, PreOncoOrders was created for the cancer clinic. It is a convenient system to preorder treatments for patients at any time before the clinical encounter. For patient safety, patient orders are tied to a 14-digit case number, their medical record number, and their name. On the first visit a patient makes to the cancer clinic, all of this information is typed in and the orders are "replayed" for the patient. If the patient's condition changes, however, the PreOncoOrders planned orders cannot be easily modified and they must be completely reentered. Another limitation is that the orders are tied to a specific date. If the day of treatment needs to be altered it is not a simple matter specifying a new date. With PreOncoOrders the patient may not have received the exact dose ordered, but this information is only recorded on paper notes and charts, not on the order-set where it would be available to help guide future orders. PreOncoOrders is not as flexible as oncologists need it to be. To allow orders to be written and modified in this way the order-set writer in OrderAssistant first needed to be modified. Order sets must be dynamic and must be able to be updated for each visit and modified for a missed appointment. With these requirements, OncoOrders was going to require a lot of development effort. Compounding that problem was a lack of funding from either the Cancer Center or the Informatics Department to get the project off the ground.

The early work was done by postdoctoral fellows in the Biomedical Informatics Department. Systems requirements were determined with regular meetings with staff from the Cancer Clinic and by having the fellows observe firsthand the work being done in the milieu of the Cancer Clinic. These meetings were well attended by staff from the Cancer Center which provided as much support as it could outside of financing the project. Clinic observers identified certain needs that were unique to the Cancer Center. One of these needs is the ability to track patients by name, location, and activity. Tracking the patients in the cancer clinic is a difficult process. The patient's first sign in at the front desk and check in for whatever appointments he or she has that day. A cancer patient could have an appointment in the clinic and one to receive a chemotherapy infusion. If a patient has an infusion appointment they must either get blood drawn for lab work at the lab, or go back to the infusion room to have samples drawn from their "tap." The infusion process can take anywhere from 30 min to 7 h for out-patient treatment. These visits must be timed with the patient's clinic visits.

Before any infusion can begin, lab values are checked for white blood cell counts, serum creatinine, and any number of other things related to the patient's health. Once the results have come back and if they have not uncovered any problems, the patient, if he or she is ready for chemotherapy, is placed in one of the infusion rooms and therapy can begin. If there are problems, the chemotherapy dose may need to be attenuated or omitted altogether. Advances in therapy are constantly changing the way care is delivered. New medications such as "Neulasta" now give the physician the ability to augment the white blood count and continue with aggressive chemotherapy in the face of declining immunocompetency. These innovations are a boon for patients but illustrate the constantly evolving nature of cancer treatment. Designing a set of systems requirements for this process is akin to hitting a moving target. By the time you have them completed, they may well be out of date.

Patients register on a sign-in sheet located in the infusion room. This alerts the nurses that the patient is ready for treatment. As soon as lab work has been returned and is in order, treatment may be initiated once treatment orders are obtained. Once the patient is signed in, his or her chart containing the orders is pulled from a large file kept in the infusion room. This chart is referred to by some as a "shadow chart" since it is only available in the cancer center and references jargon and acronyms that clinicians outside the field of oncology would have difficulty deciphering. Among the pages the chart details the treatment course to date, cumulative doses of medications received, pertinent lab data, and clinical observations. The day before the patient is scheduled to receive chemotherapy a clinical nurse specialist (Nurse Practitioner) reviews each patient's chart and treatment plan. Following the physician's treatment plan, the nurse writes medication orders that explicitly dictate the type and manner of treatment. These order sheets are placed in an accordion file for use the following day. These orders are transmitted to the pharmacy to prepare the medications for administration. When patients arrive to receive treatment nurses retrieve their order sheets from the file. If for any reason the orders were not prepared or cannot be located, the nurse must go to the patient's chart and search for the treatment plan and attempt to derive new orders. Failing that, the patient's physician must be contacted for a copy of the original orders. The same scenario may occur if a patient's orders expire, or they need modification in the orders due to change in the health of the patient. Once all the necessary paperwork has been found and a patient is found to be well enough to tolerate the treatment, infusion can begin.

Funding

Without funding available to support the development of a chemotherapy order-entry system, it was not possible to hire new employees or contract with an outside provider. It was determined that the project would be assigned to postdoctoral fellows who already had funding but needed a research project.

After a few months of working on the OncoOrders project, the first fellow decided to resign in order to pursue a residency in pathology at another institution. We were not able to interview him but we were able to learn some of his findings from a report he had produced called "OncoOrders – The Inception Phase." This report is a comprised of a very thorough analysis of Cancer Center operations and proposes a series of system requirements for OncoOrders. In this report he warned that there were a number of risks that might thwart progress on the project. He observed that each oncology service (medical oncology, surgical oncology, gynecology oncology, hematology oncology, etc.) had their own protocols and unique ways of ordering chemotherapy. Even within each service there existed "no formal policy on how chemotherapy orders are written, verified, and processed." "The 'business logic' describing how orders are handled is primarily maintained as verbal lore within the medical, nursing, and pharmacy communities." He felt that the workflow and business logic employed was "quite complex" and the work environment tended to be "chaotic" and "unpredictable." Given the size and complexity of the Cancer Center environment he felt that it would be "challenging to accurately determine the scope of the project." He was also concerned that system errors could have potentially fatal consequences. The margin for error is not very wide in a place where patients are receiving some fairly toxic medications.

After the first fellow's departure a second postdoctoral fellow inherited the project. Some further preliminary analysis was done before this second Fellow left to pursue a career in private industry. The following year a junior faculty member was brought in to oversee the project. He did not get a chance to work on it however as he was reassigned to work on another project soon after arriving. This other project had higher institutional priority and needed someone new to helm it as the current manager had accepted an offer to work at another institution.

By this time, an informatics training program had been started in the Southwest Regional Informatics department. The first class of students in the degree program, were assigned to work on the chemotherapy project as a team. There were three students assigned to the project which was treated as a master's thesis. It appeared headway was being made but this came to a sudden halt as these students were weighed down with a heavy academic course load in the second semester. After accomplishing some background work these students eventually decided to pursue other areas of research. Already having suffered from long delays, numerous changes in leadership, and little institutional support, OncoOrders was beginning to earn a reputation as an informatics quagmire. The prospective users were becoming frustrated with unfulfilled promises as well. It was realized that more resources would have to be allocated to reinvigorate the project and place it on a track to success.

The Informatics Center decided that OncoOrders would become a priority project with departmental funding beginning in 2003. This was the first time that full-time employees were hired to work on the chemotherapy project. OrderAssistant's developer and project leader each offered a small portion of their week to work on the project. William Tandy was hired as a programmer for the team. Sarah Jones, a registered nurse with clinical experience, was hired to oversee design of the project. Paul Smith was drafted in to help with the infusion room whiteboard. OrderAssistant would be adapted by the OrderAssistant team. Paul adapted the EDs whiteboard so it could be used in the Cancer Clinic.

A very-aggressive 6-month deadline was set for the deliverable prototype of OncoOrders, the order-entry system for outpatient chemotherapy treatment. Not long after the deadline was set it became apparent that the infusion room whiteboard would need to be in place and functioning before computerized order entry would be of much assistance. Coordinating the flow of patients through the clinic was the more pressing problem. Also, achieving some rapid success here would demonstrate the benefits of the system, creating "buy in" from users, and thus give the lagging OncoOrders project momentum it sorely needed.

The Whiteboard

It is important to note that the EDs whiteboard took 8 years to develop into a fully-integrated and functional system. The whiteboard went live in the ED in 2002. The whiteboard has a clean elegant interface that belies the system's complexity. It integrates information from 11 different clinical systems. Some of these "backend feeds" would remain unchanged for use in the infusion room, but many of them would need much modification. It was becoming clear that it would not be a simple task to adapt the ED whiteboard to use in the Cancer Clinic.

Another problem that beset the whiteboard team was that while the ED application performed well it ran with approximately 97% uptime. This was deemed unacceptable for the ED environment where greater than 99.9% uptime was demanded. Much of the downtime was not due to flaws in the whiteboard software itself. When any one of the 11 backend systems that feed the whiteboard data go down, the whiteboard doesn't function creating the appearance that the whiteboard itself is down. It is estimated that 20% of the downtime is due to whiteboard malfunctions. The rest of downtime is thought to be related to outside system failures. Regardless of what was causing the downtime it was decided that the ED whiteboard stability was a higher priority than the infusion room whiteboard project. The ED whiteboard team would focus solely on improving system stability until the goal of 99.9% uptime was met. At first it was anticipated that this goal could be met in a matter of a few weeks. However, weeks soon turned into months and the ED whiteboard team was still receiving requests for new functionality that needed to be added before work on the Cancer Clinic whiteboard could begin.

Despite the difficulty in getting development moving, most of the requirements of the Cancer Clinic whiteboard had been fleshed out. The whiteboard should be designed to track patients' locations during their visits. It should display relevant lab-values as soon as they are available to save nurses time from having to query StarPanel every so often for new results. Patients might have tests run outside of the clinic such as diagnostic radiology. They may also have clinical encounters outside the Cancer Clinic itself. This information would need to be continually updated so the location of the patient could be ascertained with a glance at the whiteboard. Oncology nurses complained that they wasted much of their time trying to track patients down and get them from one location to the next. Various solutions were suggested such as patient-issued magnetic swipe cards or RFID tagged bracelets that could be used to register patient location in real time.

The whiteboard modifications were originally set to be finished in March of 2004, however, this deadline could not be met, and in November of 2004 a second competing Cancer Clinic whiteboard project was started by a programmer outside the ED whiteboard group. This independent project is whimsically referred to as "Project fluoxetine" owing its name to the antidepressant more commonly known Prozac. It is hoped that this outside effort will either win out on its own merits or at least spur the ED whiteboard development team to push harder on their own development.

Order Assistant

The OrderAssistant development team already had a lot of strictly OrderAssistant related feature requests waiting to be done. Modifying the OrderAssistant to work in an outpatient clinic would require radical changes. To continue moving ahead with the order-entry system, orders and rule sets must be created for each chemotherapy treatment. Chemotherapy orders are often very complex and written for a period of 1 month to 1 year in advance. When a patient comes for treatment, the order must be evaluated based on how far along they are in the protocol, and their ability to tolerate the treatment dictated by clinical signs and results from labs drawn the day of the visit. New treatment methods and clinical trials are constantly being added; this makes adapting an order-entry system very difficult. Inpatient order-entry is simpler in that the system generally knows where to send orders by printing them out near the patient's bed location. Cancer Clinic patients' locations were not registered within the ADT system (EPIC) with that degree of accuracy. Inpatient orders are usually simple and direct without a lot of room for interpretation. Oncology differs in that orders are more conditional in nature and omit details which are left for the nurse's discretion.

With regard to billing practices another important difference is that inpatient orders do not necessarily need to be associated with an ICD9 code for reimbursement purposes. Outpatient orders require appropriate DRG/ICD9 codes be provided with each order. Without these codes the hospital or provider doesn't get paid. OrderAssistant is not set up to process these codes right now. Other changes include the ability to track cumulative doses (the actual dose the patient received which isn't always what was ordered) and track orders being sent to the pharmacy, so the chemotherapy treatment is prepared properly. This issue is further complicated by the fact that the pharmacy is in the middle of implementing a new pharmacy management system called Horizon Meds Manager. Estimates vary as to when this project will be complete. For OncoOrders to function properly, it will need to work with Horizon Meds Manager.

Evaluation

The OncoOrders project is much larger and more complicated than it was originally thought to be. When the project started, no funding and resources were provided to back it up. People were asked to add more work to their already over-crowded schedules, as a result the project continued to fail. With the increase in funding and employee hiring dedicated solely to the project, the project has a much better chance of success. The project is beginning to move forward, however, there is a lot of work left to be done. Sarah, the newest member of the team, is leaving for personal reasons and someone new must be hired to take her place. The new employee will be able to act more as a programmer now that the groundwork for the project has been laid.

The cancer center staff has always been supportive of the chemotherapy project. The nurses and physicians regularly attend meetings for the project, something that is often a problem in a project that has failed in the past. If the staff continues to be supportive, OncoOrders will be able to move ahead on its new schedule.

Potential problems still exist in the project. The timeline for the project needs to be more realistic because the original timeline did not take into account the scope of the problem. And the ED whiteboard must be up 99% of the time before it can be implemented in the cancer clinic, a barrier that will be very hard to overcome with so many systems being accessed. The order sets for the patients still need to be written and tested for safety, and the rules must be complete before the entire project can be set loose. But, by learning from the mistakes of the past, the project will be able to move ahead. The project is organized so that small chunks can be completed and both the users and the developers can see their systems moving towards completion. Unfortunately because of these past issues, the OncoOrders project will suffer from the "sins of the past." Many of the people working on the project refer to each barrier as "the curse of the OncoOrders project."

Questions

1. Should the cancer clinic have bought a stand-alone vendor system in 1998? Should they consider a vendor system now?
2. Who should contribute the funding for the project, the cancer center or the informatics department?
3. What three things should have been required for success? Explain in detail and include why you selected these three.
4. List the risks associated with this project and prioritize them. How should these risks be addressed?

13
Implementing a Computerized Triage System in the Emergency Department

Scott R. Levin, Daniel J. France, and Dominik Aronsky

Introduction

Information Technology (IT) solutions are rapidly being developed for different health care applications throughout the country's hospitals. The development and implementation of IT applications go through different phases. To successfully implement an IT application, these phases have to be merged with process re-engineering and organizational changes. The required organizational changes are critical to the overall success of IT implementation projects, but the required efforts to achieve the institutional level of commitment remain underestimated and, as a result, often cause unforeseen outcomes and implementation failures. From the very first moments of an IT implementation effort, the technological system capabilities must be tightly coupled with change processes and user involvement. Although common sense supports the idea that the IT application should support a health care provider in caring for patients, it frequently occurs that health care providers are asked to support the IT application. This may lead to the design of systems that have a lower degree of user acceptance and data integrity.

This case study reports the evolution and implementation of an IT application that transformed the process of triaging patients from a paper-based infrastructure to a computerized environment in the Emergency Department (ED) of an academic medical center in the southeast of the United States. The ED environment is challenging from an information management perspective and includes complex, time-critical tasks in situations that frequently look chaotic to an outside observer. In addition, overcrowding, a nation-wide nurse shortage, inefficiencies, and an increasingly sicker and older population contribute to challenge the ED's ability to provide high-quality health care on a daily basis. In an attempt to improve ED information management, a family of IT applications have been developed and implemented in the ED. The computerized triage application is one of these IT tools. The case study illustrates the various challenges that were encountered during the project's development life span covering the phases from early brainstorming, various prototypes and implementation attempts, to postimplementation evaluation. The currently implemented computerized triage application is described and conclusions are drawn about why specific attempts at developing a computerized triage application were aborted and why the final attempt was successful.

L. Einbinder et al. (eds.), *Transforming Health Care Through Information: Case Studies*, Health Informatics, DOI 10.1007/978-1-4419-0269-6_13, © Springer Science+Business Media, LLC 2010

The Institution and IT Environment

The setting of the case study is an academic, tertiary, Level I trauma center serving a primarily urban population. The medical center fosters a fairly advanced and progressive IT environment supporting the management of patient information. Over the last decade, the medical center has invested considerable efforts to build a broad portfolio of IT applications that would improve the quality of patient care through the intelligent use of informatics applications. These applications are designed to allow health care providers to combine their clinical decision making skills with computer-delivered health information at the point of patient care. These applications are a combination of vendor-based and in-house developed systems. A strong interface among various applications acts as the "informatics glue" allowing a relatively high level of integration that supports the transparent flow of information. Among the various systems, we briefly introduce the three applications that are relevant to this case study: computerized patient record system, the provider order entry system, and the ED information system.

StarPanel is the institution's longitudinal computerized patient record system, which acts as the main data repository and aggregates a diverse set of clinical information such as demographic information, lab results, radiology reports, discharge summaries, order summaries, anatomic pathology, physician notes and letters.[1] StarPanel integrates data from multiple sources and allows users to manage clinical information from the perspective of a specific patient or from an entire patient population. The information in StarPanel is available through a Web browser and may be accessed using the numerous shared workstations within the medical center. StarPanel includes a strong communication component through message baskets that allows provider teams to manage the flow of patient information.[2]

WizOrder is the institution's computerized provider order entry system, which is implemented on all hospital units (including the ED) for the management of patients' orders.[3,4] WizOrder includes a rich and intelligent decision-support mechanism that helps providers during the decision-making process. Patient-specific information involving allergies and recent laboratory and test results are available within the system. WizOrder also incorporates intelligent advisory systems, access to clinical literature and evidence-based order sets, which provide an advanced information management infrastructure at the point of care.

StarPanel and WizOrder have been instrumental in reducing medical errors and providing improved quality of care to patients. An example includes the next-day contact of all patients with a Vioxx prescription when reports surfaced about heart-related side effects potentially caused by the medication.[5] This was accomplished through StarPanel's population-based search capabilities. Another example includes the reduction of medication errors in the pediatric intensive care unit.[6] In addition to the institutions' core IT applications, several units have developed more specialized IT applications that support more specialized tasks, e.g., the operating room, the outpatient clinics, or the ED.

The ED includes pediatric and adult units, which provide care to more than 85,000 patients annually. Information management in an ED environment is complex and characterized by information snippets, frequent interruptions, multitasking, and periods of increased workloads.[7-9] It is not surprising that the ED environment is suspected of having one of the highest rates of medical errors.[10] Information management using IT applications may contribute to an improved and safer ED environment. Vanderbilt's

ED operation is supported by an ED information system.[11,12] The ED information system leverages the institution's general IT applications, such as the Admit-Discharge-Transfer system, StarPanel, and WizOrder, and integrates them with ED-specific IT applications.

The core of the ED information system infrastructure includes an advanced computerized whiteboard system that tracks patients through their encounter in the ED. The whiteboard serves as the primary point of entry for most information management needs. It provides detailed, patient-specific tracking information from the time of ED registration to discharge, and displays ED operational statistics related to patient flow, occupancy levels and waiting-room queues. In addition, the ED information system provides a framework for alerts concerning the availability of lab results, radiology reports, consult services, etc. The whiteboard system is integrated with StarPanel and WizOrder giving health care providers transparent and easy access to patient information. The ED whiteboard is displayed on two touch-sensitive, 60-in. plasma screens and on all ED workstations. The system is browser-based allowing access throughout the hospital. The ED information system is a very effective information management tool that supports all staff involved in patient care, such as physicians, consultants, nurses, technicians, registration staff, environmental services, administrators, etc. for clinical, operational, educational, quality improvement, and research tasks.

Parallel to these real-time capabilities is the ability of the ED information system to systematically store and time stamp all information that is being entered by staff. This information is stored in the institution's enterprise data warehouse, which provides a very rich arena for analysis and retrospective research. StarPanel, WizOrder and the ED information system comprise the core IT infrastructure available in the ED. In the ED's attempt to gradually move into a primarily computer-based patient care environment and to streamline the flow of information, the ED has invested in efforts to develop its computerized triage application. The computerized triage application was envisioned as a computer-based and integrated triage application that supports the ED triage team in making appropriate ED resource allocation early during a patient's ED encounter.

Triage Basics

The main purpose of ED triage is to prioritize incoming patients and quickly identify those patients who must be seen immediately.[13] The military has applied triage systems, which have been introduced, adopted, and refined by civilian hospitals since the late 1960s. Changes in the health care delivery system during the 1950s and 1960s created a large increase in the amount of patients presenting to EDs throughout the country. This increase in volume was a result of many patients using the ED for less-severe or nonemergent health problems. Federal law determines that each patient presenting to the ED must be evaluated through a medical screening exam by a physician.[14] The triage process helps EDs to prioritize their efforts under frequently occurring overload situations.

The basis of triage is an acuity scale. Each patient is assigned an acuity value based upon specific criteria. Currently, several different types of ED triage systems are used. The different triage systems apply various scales that may range from 2 to 5 distinct levels (Table 13.1). In 2001, the Emergency Nurses Association (ENA) surveyed 1,380 ED managers representing 27% of all EDs in the United States to find out which triage acuity scales were being used.[15]

TABLE 13.1. Examples of triage acuity systems (adapted from 13).

2 Levels	3 Levels	4 Levels	5 Levels
Emergent	Emergent	Life-threatening	Resuscitation
Nonemergent	Urgent	Emergent	Emergent
	Nonurgent	Urgent	Urgent
		Nonurgent	Nonurgent
			Referred

They found that 69% of EDs use a 3-level system, 12% a 4-level system, and 3% a 5-level system. Inherent challenges to triage systems include the lack of differentiation among patients, and limitations in internal and external instrument reliability resulting in poor reproducibility and large variances. Until recently, triage systems have not been developed using a systematic approach. With the development and dissemination of the 5-level Emergency Severity Index (ESI), the Emergency Nursing Association and the American College of Emergency Physicians have recognized the need for acuity scale standardization.[13] The two professional organizations support the adoption of the ESI 5-level triage system.[16,17] The ESI is currently the best-researched triage instrument, demonstrating reliability and validity.[13,18,19] Other currently used 5-level triage systems include the Australian Triage Scale,[20,21] the Manchester Triage Scale[22] and the Canadian Triage and Acuity Scale.[23-25] The ESI differs from the other systems as it incorporates the prediction of patient resource consumption. The Agency for Healthcare Research and Quality (AHRQ) has adopted the ESI as the most beneficial triage scale available for EDs in the U.S.[13] Figure 13.1 displays the basic algorithm for triaging patients using the ESI.

The Vanderbilt ED moved from a 4-level acuity to the ESI 5-level scale in March of 2004. One of the limitations of the ESI remains the use of "weasel words," i.e., terms that are not well defined and impossible to perform a computerized evaluation.[26] An example is the ESI level 2 criteria of "high-risk situation" (Fig. 13.1). Although the ESI manual provides some guidance for interpretation, the concept remains vague and difficult to computerize. Despite these challenges, the ED developed a computerized triage application that guides triage nurses in assigning an ESI level in an effort to increase the inter-rater reliability and validity of the process. In the following sections, the implementation experiences of transitioning from a paper-based to a computerized triage infrastructure is described. This will include the pertinent aspects of introducing a new application in a rapidly paced environment, the encountered challenges and how they were finally overcome.

An overall timeline of ED systems implantation is displayed in Fig. 13.2, and helps understand the temporal relationships among the various systems and among the different triage implementation approaches.

Paper-Based Triage Process

Up until March of 2004, triage documentation in both the pediatric and adult ED was completed using a paper form (Fig. 13.3). At the registration desk, the clerk would sign the patient in by filling in the header information on the triage form (Fig. 13.3). Several additional paper forms were added to the paper chart. Next, the triage nurse would

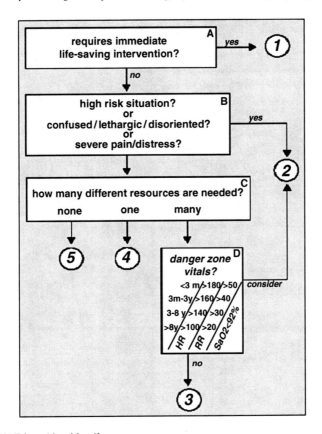

FIG. 13.1. ESI Triage Algorithm.[13]

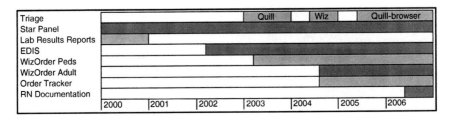

FIG. 13.2. Timeline for the various computerized applications that were introduced to the Vanderbilt Medical Center IT environment.

call the next patient to be triaged based upon the presenting chief complaint noted. The triage nurse would assess the patient's illness by asking a series of questions, taking vital signs and completing a short assessment (Fig. 13.3). At the end of the triage process, the triage nurse would select and record an International Classification of Diseases (ICD9-CM) code for the patient's chief complaint from a list available at the triage station. At the same time, the triage nurse would assign a final acuity value.

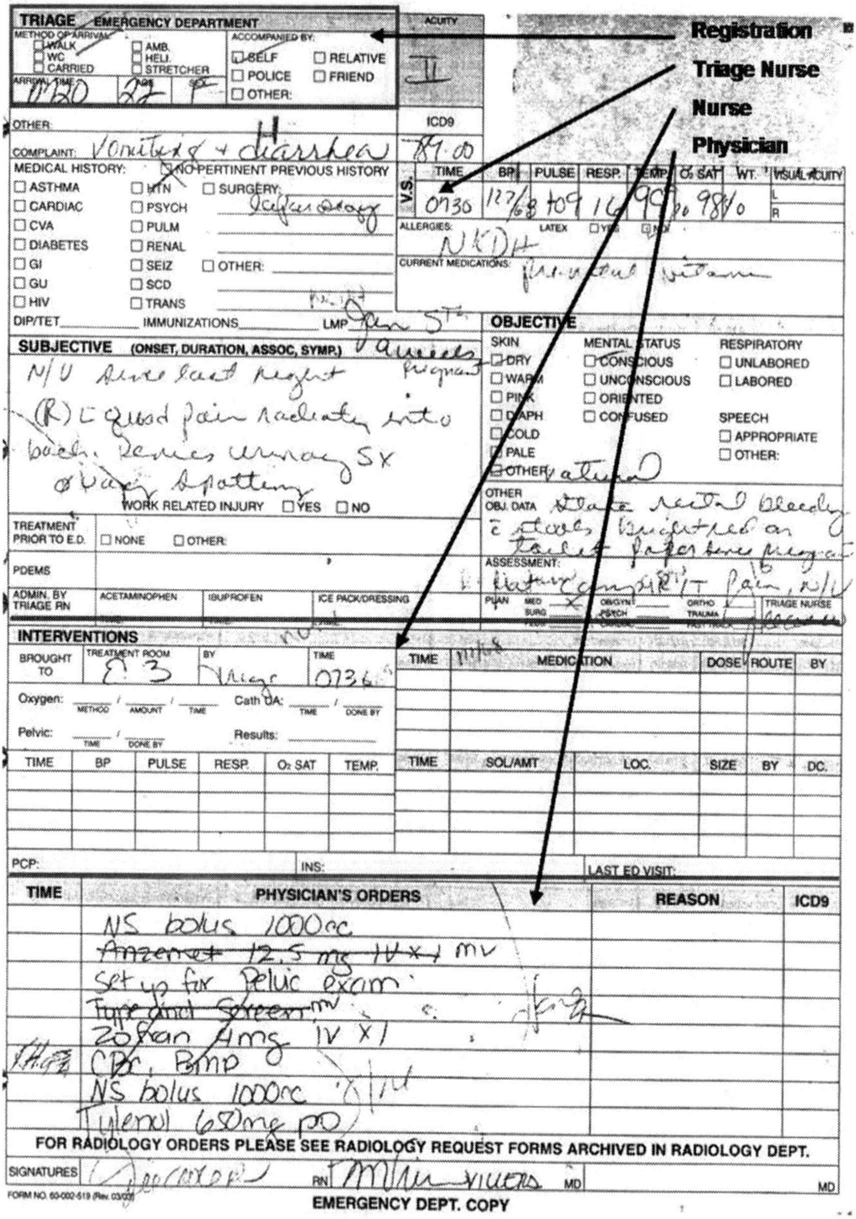

FIG. 13.3. Paper triage form included in patient chart. Each section was completed by the staff member labeled as a patient moved through the different stages of ED care.

Next, the triage nurse would direct the patient to a bed or escort the patient back to the waiting room. The bed placement decision was made based upon bed availability and the clinical status of the patient. The triage form was clipped to the patient's ED chart and remained there from registration to discharge. After the patient was moved into a treatment bed, the patient chart was placed in a basket located on the wall next to the patient's room. The nurses, technicians and physicians would then continue to fill out their section of the form as the patient was evaluated, treated, and discharged from the ED (Fig. 13.3).

This triage process was effective, but relatively slow and suffered from the many shortcomings intrinsic to paper-based systems. Illegible documentation, use of nonstandard abbreviations, and incomplete data capture contributed to inefficient information management and could lead to confusion, medical errors, and potentially adverse events. Clinicians were put into situations where they were guessing what was recorded on the form. If vital signs were unreadable, they would need to be taken again. Questions asked during triage would be repeated further down the line of patient care. Another shortcoming of the paper-based system was the paper itself. An average of 200 patients were seen daily, each having 7–10 forms making up their complete ED chart. Organizing this large quantity of paper flowing through the often hectic ED proved challenging. Forms could easily come up missing forcing providers to devote time toward searching for misplaced charts or recreating permanently lost charts. Then, following a patient's discharge the paper forms must be stored, managed and easily retrievable. The paper-based process exhibited several problems that needed to be addressed and provided an opportunity for improvement. The need for improved documentation practices and the desire to streamline the information management process prompted a small team to examine the potential benefits of a computerized triage application.

Initial Triage IT Development

The preliminary steps in creating a computerized triage application went underway in the summer of 2003. A team composed of two experienced nurses (information system consultants) and a biomedical informaticist began to brainstorm the most effective computerized triage application development pathway. This core team held reoccurring meetings with the ED director (a physician) and nurse manager to gain a high-level understanding of how the new system would be used. The nurse consultant then began to shadow several of the triage nurses to understand the details of the paper-based triage process. The information obtained from the meetings and observations was used to determine a minimal set of system requirements. It was also discussed whether the new system should be based on:

(a) Adapting an already existing information technology
(b) Developing a new application
(c) Purchasing a system from an outside vendor

The last option was quickly dismissed, as there was no vendor that offered a computerized triage application product that included the ESI algorithm. After weighing the other two options and discussing available resources for programming efforts, a decision was made. The team would examine the potential of Vanderbilt's existing controlled data capture application (Quill).

Quill

Quill[27] is a frame-based, general purpose data entry tool that utilizes a controlled vocabulary to capture clinical information. The clinical documentation system has already been implemented and is in use in the Cardiology Department. The system was developed and is maintained by the academic medical center's informatics department, and includes two components. A controlled vocabulary forms the foundation of the application. A graphical user interface (GUI) allows the user to enter data that are linked to the vocabulary components. The application provides customizable templates, which are aggregations of elements from the structured vocabulary. Existing templates from any department can be easily retrieved and modified for an individual user's needs. The captured data are stored in the application database and also transformed into easily readable clinical notes that are sent to StarPanel, the computerized patient record system. Previous reports, e.g., from a patient's previous visit, are retrievable and can be updated with information from the current visit. The application's GUI is shown in Fig. 13.4, and follows a vertical-oriented outline, similar to a tree-structure that can be expanded and collapsed.

The information system consultants met several times with the triage nurses and ED managers to refine the content and layout. The process incorporated most of the information from the paper form (Fig. 13.4). The Quill application was not able to easily

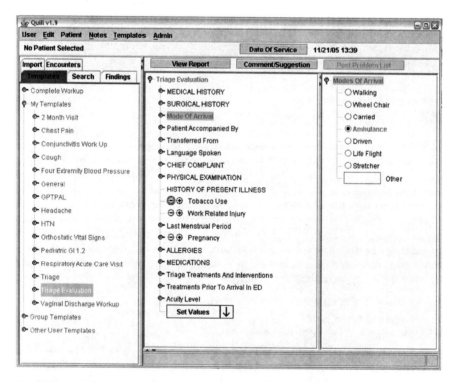

Fig. 13.4. Quill application GUI. Based on a vertical-oriented tree structure in which bulleted sections may be expanded in the left-most and middle window. The data are entered in the right-most window where the selected section is displayed.

TABLE 13.2. Quill application pro/con evaluation.

Pros	Cons
Structured documentation tool	Could not do calculations
Useful controlled vocabulary	Hard to integrate with other existing IT tools
Data storage methods were in place	Patient selection in GUI was very tedious
Proven useful in Cardiology Department	GUI was unintuitive
Capable of generating error messages	Inputting data was too time consuming
Relatively inexpensive	Steep learning curve
Easily provided printable reports	
Existing implementation and support team	
Scalable solution	

incorporate several key features that a successful computerized triage application would need. The team created the main frame of the application including only the basic features that were easiest to implement. The more time-consuming and difficult features would be added at a later point when more programming resources became available. When the system was demonstrated to the triage nurses, it was found to be unintuitive, not user friendly, and difficult to navigate in triage. The perception was that the tool would not be able to meet the needs of the fast-paced ED environment. It is recommended that a comprehensive triage assessment be made on a patient in 2–5 min.[28] It was felt that the Quill application would have prohibited this from occurring. There was an excessive amount of point-and-click and it seemed to take longer than completing its primary competitor, the original paper form. The system was further analyzed by the informaticist, the nurses and ED managers. A pro/con evaluation of the system can be seen in Table 13.2. The system was known to have a steeper initial learning curve, but that may become more efficient once the user was familiar with the interface. Although progress and further improvements were made, the GUI ultimately proved to be the application's downfall. After only a few months, the system was determined to be impractical for the ED triage process and abandoned. The system never went live in the ED and at this point the team decided to explore other means of creating a computerized triage application.

WizOrder

With the implementation of computerized provider order entry in the ED, the need to document patients' allergies and weights moved to the forefront. Capturing weights was particularly important to the pediatric ED where weight-based medication dosing is critical. The ongoing programming resource limitations experienced by the ED information system team, prompted the order entry development team to take on the task of designing and implementing a computerized triage application. The significance of having patients' weights and allergies available during an ordering session propelled the team to incorporate a computerized triage application in WizOrder. The order entry development team was comprised of a system support staff member, the manager of the pediatric ED, several pediatric nurses, the director of the adult and pediatric ED and several members of the Biomedical Informatics Department. Compared to the previous attempt, a significantly bigger collaborative effort was put forth in order to get a computerized triage application off the ground. The highest priority of the newly assembled team was to integrate weight and allergy information collected at triage into WizOrder. This would allow the provider order entry system to check the appropriateness of medication orders. An alert message would pop up in WizOrder when an order with an unsafe medication or unsafe medication dosage was placed. This was believed to be a potentially critical medication error reduction strategy within the ED. Over a 4-month period the team began to develop a triage application within WizOrder.

A biomedical informatics postdoctoral fellow spearheaded the application development. There were initial concerns from the ED information system development team that WizOrder was not designed to support documentation, storage, and reporting of clinical information. In addition, the browser-based environment had considerable GUI limitations. Despite the concerns, the development efforts were pushed forward. The development team met regularly with the triage nurses and ED managers to gain a thorough understanding of the system requirements. As before, the nurses resisted change and requested a GUI that was identical to the paper triage form they were used to. This GUI, which successfully replicated the form, can be seen in Fig. 13.5. The more intense development efforts resulted in a GUI that was liked by the pediatric users. The full application was tested and demonstrated to the triage nurses. The application was usually launched before the users arrived at the demonstration sessions. Because of this, the users did not realize that getting to the start of the embedded triage documentation required a substantial amount of time. The user must sign in, launch the order session and then identify and open the triage application. In relation to the triage documentation process, the application initiation process and to get to the point where triage data entry could begin was time-consuming. It was determined that it took over 30 seconds to completely launch the application. This was frustrating for the ED triage nurses and perceived as an inefficient process for the high volume of patients seen daily in the ED. Several other limitations, mostly related to usability, further hindered the user group to buy-in to the application. One limitation involved the user's inability to tab through the many fields that are required to submit the document. In addition, the incorporation of the ESI algorithm and several other perceived benefits were not achievable within the order entry framework.

A pro/con evaluation of this system can be seen in Table 13.3. The application's inability to launch and the system limitations that arose during GUI development, forced the project to be terminated shortly before the planned go-live date. WizOrder did not provide the structure necessary to create an effective computerized triage application. Forcing a computerized triage application within this framework was not an appropriate solution.

Designing the Current System

Two abortive attempts at implementing a computerized triage application left the ED user group disappointed, and the ED information system team and the development team discouraged. Despite the invested time and effort with two approaches, the ED information system team and the ED user group remained positive to find a working solution. It was felt that the two initial approaches had many positive aspects, but that the ED group had to commit to compromises that had a considerable impact on the triage process. The desire for an "ideal" system increased even more.

After obtaining external funding, subsidized by the institution, the existing ED information system development team was able to successfully design and introduce a computerized

Pediatric ED Triage Form

Method of arrival: ____

Accompanied by: ____   Other: ____

Medical record number ____   Encounter number ____

Patient name ____   Patient sex: **female**

Patient age: **28 years**   Arrival time: **04/08/04 10:13**

Initial patient complaint: **PAIN**

Acuity ____   PCP: ____

Transfer: Y N   From: ____

Onset of illness: ____   Time of injury: ____

Current history: ____

Immunizations: UID NUID

LMP: ____   Pregnant: Y N

Pain:

Y N

Unable to determine

Scale ____   Score ____

Consolable: Y N

Tx. prior to ED: None

Vital Signs: Patient crying: Y N

TIME SBP DBP PULSE RESP TEMP Method

WT(kg) RW(kg) O2SAT Visual Acuity L R

Comments: ____   Unable to obtain

Medical History:

- None
- ADHD
- Asthma
- Cancer
- Cardiac
- Dev. Delay

- Diabetes
- GI
- GU
- Hiv
- Hydroceph
- Intubation

- PICU
- NICU
- Renal
- SCD
- Psych
- Pulm

- Surgery ____
- Premature ____ wks
- Seiz
- Transp.
- VP Shunt
- Other

- TB Exposure
- Bld. and body fluid
- Resp. isolation

Current Medications: See attached sheet None

Medication	Route	Dose	Freq	Last Given

PATHWAY:
- Laceration
- Ear Pain
- Sore Troat
- Knee
- Asthma
- Trauma Note
- Critical Event
- Eye
- Ankle
- Dental

AIRWAY:
- WNL
- Patent
- Stridor
- Injured
- Intubated
- Drooling
- Compromised
- Nasal Congestion
- Other: ____

BREATHING:
- WNL
- Clear
- Equal
- Rales
- Crackles
- Wheezing
- Labored
- Diminished
- Other: ____

CIRCULATION:
- WNL Dry
- Pink Diaphoretic
- Pale Other ____
- Jaundice
- Mottled
- Cyanosis
- Capillary refill: ____
- Membranes: Moist Dry
- Heart Rate: Reg. Irreg.

ACTIVITY:
- Playful Unresponsive
- Lethargic Limp
- Listless Other: ____
- Alert
- Responds to verbal
- Responds to pain
- Age Appropriate: Y N
- Baseline: Y N
- PERRL: Y N

ABDOMEN:
- WNL
- Soft
- Nontender
- Tender
- Distended
- Rigid
- Redness
- Ecchymosis
- Other: ____

BACK/CHEST:
- WNL
- Soft
- Nontender
- Tender
- Redness
- Ecchymosis
- Deformity
- Edema
- Other: ____

HEAD/NECK:
- WNL
- Fontanel: ____
- Swelling: ____
- Redness: ____
- Ecchymosis: ____
- Other: ____

EXTREMITIES:
- WNL

  PULSES   MOVEMENT
- R.Arm Pres Abs Dec Yes No Wounds/Deform ____
- L.Arm Pres Abs Dec Yes No Wounds/Deform ____
- R Leg Pres Abs Dec Yes No Wounds/Deform ____
- L Leg Pres Abs Dec Yes No Wounds/Deform ____

PSYCHIATRIC:
- Not Applicable
- Calm Hallucinations
- Cooperative Auditory
- Agitated Visual
- Sullen Combative
- Suicidal Ideation
- Homicidal Ideation
- Non-Communicative
- Informant: ____

Room: ____   Time: ____   By: ____

Report to: ____   Time: ____

Assessment: ____

Allergies: ____   No Known Allergies

SUBMIT TRIAGE FORM   **CANCEL TRIAGE FORM**

Fig. 13.5. WizOrder triage application GUI. Data was input through check boxes, pull down menus and free text input boxes. The major limitation of the GUI involved the user's inability to tab through input fields.

triage application into the ED. The team included the standing ED information system team members from the adult and pediatric ED (managers, nurses, registration staff, educators, physicians, etc.), the developers and a biomedical informaticist. There was a significant increase in time and effort devoted to developing the current computerized triage application in comparison to the two previous attempts. The initial task was to

TABLE 13.3. WizOrder application pro/con evaluation.

Pros	Cons
Incorporated weights and allergies	Not designed to be a documentation system
Already integrated with order entry system	Could not run at the same time as StarPanel
Performed simple calculations	Took over 30 s to launch
Low learning curve	Could not print
User were familiar with user interface	Could not tab through fields
	Not retrievable for reporting
	Limited user interface capabilities
	Unable to easily integrate ESI instrument

step back, and completely question and re-evaluate the entire triage process and, with it the triage documentation. The need for some level of process re-engineering was obvious. High-level discussions on what drives the triage process eventually translated into more detailed discussions about which specific data elements needed to be collected. Several meetings between members of the team with clinical expertise occurred in order to revise the data set that was going to be collected at triage. Only information that contributes to a triage decision was incorporated. All other irrelevant informations being collected were discarded, or moved to the nurse assessment process. This was done in an effort to shorten triage assessment time. The re-evaluation process also included data requirements from the Joint Commission on Accreditation of Health care Organizations (JCAHO), an independent, not-for-profit organization that sets nationwide standards for quality and safety within health care. The paper triage form did not capture all of the required data elements proposed by JCAHO. The computerized triage application project provided the team with an ideal opportunity to create a JCAHO compliant triage process. The goal of the computerized triage application was to include the new JCAHO data collection requirements and any other data that the team felt was pertinent to collect at triage. In addition, ED triage-specific algorithms would be included in the computerized triage application to increase inter-rater reliability, validity and time efficiency of the triage process. Many of the experienced nurses questioned that a detailed initial nurse assessment was not necessary at triage and opposed discarding many data variables. The reasons were familiarity with the elements on the paper-based form, and the uncertainty of how this would affect patient care at a vulnerable stage of the patient's ED encounter. With the ED managers, nurse educators, physicians, and some nurses' combined efforts and help, enough momentum was built to initiate and support this major change in documentation.

The ESI triage algorithm was being used in the ED as of March 2003. The team decided that the new computerized triage application should incorporate the ESI algorithm as a decision-guiding mechanism for the nurses when choosing an appropriate acuity level for a patient. This is desirable because a computerized decision support tool has proven to increase inter-rater reliability amongst nurses.[28] An ED in Canada compared triage evaluations by nurses using a computerized decision tool with nurses using the traditional memory-based approach. In addition to increasing inter-rater agreement, this research team was also able to mitigate a down-triaging drift that had been prevalent prior to the introduction of the decision support tool. In addition, new requirements concerning the integration of existing data elements from the Admit-Discharge-Transfer system, StarPanel and the ED information system were issued to eliminate redundant data entry and improve the functionality of the application. The exact specifications and requirements for the new computerized triage application had been developed. At this point, it was recognized that ED triage is a unique process; thus, the newly created computerized triage application infrastructure may have limited scalability and may not be of any benefit to other hospital units. However, each data element was examined for availability in the institution's information sources in order to achieve a high level of data integration and data sharing.

The desire for better data integration and data sharing steered the ED information system team toward the decision to use the controlled data capture infrastructure provided by Quill. The computerized triage application would be able to benefit from its ability to generate free text and clinical notes. This infrastructure would also allow the capture of weight and allergy information. The GUI would be browser-based similar to the other ED information system components, which would increase user adoption. The ED information system team also agreed to develop and provide the users with a structured reporting environment, which was absent from both previous attempts and was a critical element to the ED management. In addition, the ESI algorithm was computerized and additional logic was implemented. This logic was developed to help the user to quickly peruse the interface and enter the appropriate information easily. Examples of the user supporting logic include:

(a) The implementation of a pregnancy wheel for determining gestational age in pregnant women
(b) The selection of the appropriate pain scale (different for pediatric and adult patients)
(c) Capturing and recording coded chief complaints
(d) Providing the documentation for verifying a patient's identity as required by JCAHO
(e) Age-guided immunization documentation, which differs for pediatric and adult patients

Incorporation of the current medications, allergy information, and health maintenance information directly from StarPanel proved to be an invaluable time-saver and improved the accuracy of documentation within the ED. The triage specific logic and the well-integrated data elements improved the usability of the computerized triage application and the reliability of the triage process. A significant effort was made to incorporate both the adult and pediatric requirements within the same application, which resulted in an application that was perceived well by the user community.

After 8 months of development, testing, and refinement, the computerized triage application went live in June 2005 in both the pediatric and adult ED. User training was completed by ED staff members with a minimal amount of effort. ED management developed policy documents that governed the new triage application. After training was complete, the ED management and nurse users were eager to employ the computerized triage application for triaging all patients, including critically ill patients. The users found the application quick, intuitive, easy to use and helpful. The GUI of the current application is displayed in Fig. 13.6. A more thorough pro/con evaluation of the new system can be seen in Table 13.4.

This was the first successful attempt at implementing a computerized triage application. Throughout the development stages, the ED user team always recognized how the IT infrastructure could be utilized to their advantage. The ED-computerized triage application currently incorporates challenging tasks that are only accomplished at a few EDs. Some of the unique features include the availability of:

(a) A computerized ESI algorithm
(b) Screening of all patients for domestic violence
(c) Documentation of vaccination history in an ED setting

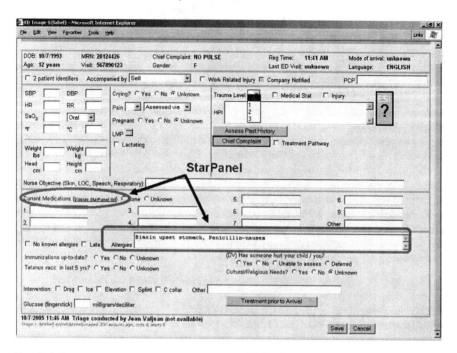

Fig. 13.6. Browser-based GUI created for the current computerized triage application. The GUI overlies the Quill documentation system which uses a controlled vocabulary to capture clinical information. The highlighted regions represent locations where data elements (current medications and allergies) from StarPanel are integrated into the GUI.

TABLE 13.4. Current computerized triage application pro/con evaluation.

Pros	Cons
User-friendly GUI	More expensive development
Provides for quick data entry	Longer development phase
Pulls medication and allergy information from StarPanel	Complex integration issues during development phase
Fully integrated with StarPanel and EDIS	Limited scalability
Structured documentation tool	
Used existing infrastructure of controlled vocabulary	
Data storage and reporting methods were in place	
Computerization of ESI algorithm	
Included JCAHO required documentation	
Capable of generating error messages	
Assigning ICD9 code for chief complaints	
Provides printable reports	
Time stamping triage process	
Data sharing	
Additional capture of billing information	

(d) Capturing the time spent on triage documentation

(e) Screening for cultural/religious needs at the point-of entry

A triage summary page is displayed after the documentation is saved. The page will alert the user to initiate important tasks such as ordering an electrocardiogram for patients with acute coronary syndrome or remind the triage nurse to contact an attending physician if critical vital signs were captured. The triage summary page also provides the infrastructure to implement specific guidelines such as prompting the user to ask additional questions, as may be required for SARS screening. In addition, a current research study sends a notification to the provider order entry system for patients who were determined to be eligible for pneumococcal vaccination. The provider order entry system will then prompt the physician that the patient may be eligible for pneumococcal vaccination at which point the vaccination order can be completed with a single action. Once the user has completed the triage documentation, a triage report is sent to StarPanel and the ED whiteboard application receives the patient's chief complaint, the ESI acuity level, and domestic violence screening information.

Analysis of Implementation Aspects

This version of the computerized triage application was successful because it directly addressed many of the problems that the previous systems exhibited. The GUI is intuitive and user-friendly. The system is fully integrated with the ED information system and StarPanel. Within seconds, the application is easily launched directly from the interfaced ED whiteboard system. Clicking on a name of a registered patient on the ED whiteboard interface will launch the computerized triage application with the correct identifying information already displayed. The computerized triage application automatically integrates medications documented in StarPanel's problem list. Allergy and immunization data from the problem list are directly passed to the computerized triage application interface (labeled in Fig. 13.6). This allows the ED triage nurse to verify allergies with previous knowledge, which is an easier and more informed way of capturing these pertinent data.

The new computerized triage application was designed to have several decision support elements incorporated. The computerized triage application uses some simple logic to assist the triage nurses in assigning an acuity level on the ESI scale through incorporating data elements from the patient's age, presenting chief complaint and vital sign fields. The triage nurse still has the ability to override the system and assign a different value, if desired; however, a brief explanation of this action must be typed into the override field. Analysis of appropriate overrides may contribute to a better understanding of potential limitations of the ESI instrument. The computerized triage application also time stamps the start and end of triage documentation. Nurse triage times may be tracked and analyzed, and they are currently used for quality improvement efforts in the ED.

The advantageous features of the system are countered by a few drawbacks, primarily the short delay for printing, WizOrder integration, and scalability. The application is able to relay a text report to StarPanel, which may be printed and added to the patient's paper chart. The user must wait for the triage report to become available in StarPanel before printing can occur. This is not ideal; however the report usually becomes available to the nurse within 10 seconds. WizOrder integration is the major drawback of the system. The current computerized triage application collects patient's weight and allergy information and sends these elements to the patient's medical record in free text format. Relaying these critical data elements to the provider order entry system has not yet been accomplished, primarily because many different IT systems have become involved. Although a solution is imminent, it remains important to realize that one of the most critically perceived goals of the computerized triage application has not been accomplished by any of the three implementation efforts. Using this information in the order entry system is currently an important short-term goal of the ED information system team. The final drawback involves the limited scalability and reusability of the chosen approach. This disadvantage was known at the onset of the project. However, the uniqueness of the problem required an equally unique solution, so the scalability issue was rendered unavoidable and offset by the many advantages of the current system.

System Evaluation

The team has completed the data collection for an evaluation of the computerized triage application. An observational study assessed the tasks involved with triaging a patient before and after the implementation of the computerized triage application. The analysis included 21 hours of observation in the pre- and 21 hours during the postimplementation phase of the project. A task-analysis was conducted in order to determine the amount of time triage nurses spent triaging specific patients. The triage times recorded from the observation will be compared to the triage times recorded by the computerized triage application to assess the validity of the computerized time stamps. System data analysis and user surveys have been conducted to determine the effectiveness of the computerized triage application. Feedback from these studies will guide future improvements to the computerized triage application as well as the entire triage process.

Discussion

The eventual success of a computerized triage application did not come until 2½ years after the initial goal was set. The IT environment had been changing significantly throughout the course of the project. Figure 13.2 illustrates the transient IT environment in relation to the development of the computerized triage application. These environmental changes controlled the direction of the project. Initially, a computerized triage application was needed to eliminate the shortcomings of a paper-based system. The potential improvements of moving from a paper-based to computerized system were addressed throughout the duration of the project. A quick deployment involving the use of an already established system, Quill, was explored. The system was designed for documentation and appeared to be a logical and inexpensive solution. There were very few recognized problems until the users became involved. The triage nurses resisted and the application was determined to be impractical. A critical system component arose when WizOrder was introduced into the pediatric ED. Importing weight and allergy information into WizOrder became the fundamental goal of the system. The enthusiasm behind providing WizOrder with critical information from triage steered the incarnation of computerized triage application development. This spurred the developers into trying to modify an existing infrastructure to support a task for which the system was not designed for. An attempt at incorporating a documentation component within a provider order entry system was made. Like the initial Quill attempt, the users finally deemed the system unusable in the actual ED setting.

The WizOrder application came very close to actual implementation. The limitations present, when creating a GUI in Quill and WizOrder, prohibited the respected systems from ever going live. Although some of these limitations were known, the project was still forced ahead.

The last successful attempt coupling the Quill vocabulary infrastructure with a user-friendly browser-based interface provided a feasible and eventually successful implementation approach. The flexibility to develop a GUI that was able to support the user's requests, while integrating the re-engineered triage process, proved invaluable during the development phase. The relatively flexible GUI was able to overlay the Quill infrastructure which had several advantages involving a controlled vocabulary. The current computerized triage application was the only attempt at using a system that satisfied both the users' and the developers' needs. In addition, the level of achieved integration with other systems was a critical factor for success. Developers were initially consumed with attempting to modify existing systems that were not designed for the unique needs of a computerized triage application. When the team recognized that a unique task required a unique tool, success was realized. What became particularly unique about this task was the dynamic and fast-paced environment of the ED users. The time length of the project from conception to implementation may have been shortened significantly had user needs been held principal to any other system goals that the developers had in mind.

Several other factors led the final computerized triage application to success and the other applications to failure. A comparison of the three systems can be seen in Table 13.5 below. The major difference in the usability of Quill-browser is highlighted by the good marks in the user-technological category. Other major differences can be seen within the support category. A successful application was unable to be created until the support for it was ample. The typical trade off between cost and quality is also demonstrated in Table 13.5.

Table 13.5. Comparison of the characteristics of the three computerized triage applications approaches.

	Quill	WizOrder	Current computerized triage application
Technological			
User			
GUI	+	++	+++
Ease of data capture	+	+	+++
Ease of reporting	++	+	++
Developer			
Level of integration	+	++	+++
Scalability	+++	+	++
Available infrastructure	+++	++	++
Support			
Financial	+	++	+++
Management	+	++	+++
Personnel	+	++	+++
Cost			
Development cost	+	++	+++
Maintenance cost	+	+	+

+ = poor, ++ = average, +++ = good

The current computerized triage application has been a success in the ED. There are some minor shortcomings of the system, but further efforts are being put forth to provide solutions. A thorough evaluation of the system is the next step. There has been much progress made in the area of data collection; however, an analysis of this data remains future work. Continuously improving the system based on these findings is still an objective of the current computerized triage application development team. The growing phases of the project demonstrated some fundamental keys to the success of an IT system:

(1) The involvement of users in the early development stages and holding their feedback paramount
(2) Moving from a paper-based to a computerized process provides an opportunity for or may require process re-engineering
(3) Obtaining a high level of managerial, financial and personnel support before an IT project is undertaken

If either of these actions is not executed, then the IT system has a strong likelihood of remaining in a developmental stage. The team realized this on their third attempt at creating a computerized triage application. The result was a very useful IT system that has improved the process of delivering health care within the ED.

References

1. Jirjis J, Patel NR, Aronsky D, Lorenzi N, Giuse D. Seeing stars: the creation of a core clinical support informatics product. *Int J Healthc Technol Manag.* 2003;5(3/4/5):284-295.
2. Giuse DA. Supporting communication in an integrated patient record system. AMIA Annu Symp Proc. 2003:1065.
3. Neilson EG, Johnson KB, Rosenbloom ST, et al. The impact of peer management on test-ordering behavior. *Ann Intern Med.* 2004;141(3):196-204.
4. Miller RA, Waitman LR, Chen S, Rosenbloom ST. The anatomy of decision support during inpatient care provider order entry (CPOE): empirical observations from a decade of CPOE experience at Vanderbilt. *J Biomed Inform.* 2005;38(6):469-485.
5. Oberholzer-Gee F, Inamdar SN. Merck's recall of rofecoxib – a strategic perspective. *N Engl J Med.* 2004;351(21):2147-2149.
6. Potts AL, Barr FE, Gregory DF, Wright L, Patel NR. Computerized physician order entry and medication errors in a pediatric critical care unit. *Pediatrics.* 2004;113:59-63.
7. Feied CF, Smith MS, Handler JA, Kanhouwa M. Emergency medicine can play a leadership role in enterprise-wide clinical information systems. *Ann Emerg Med.* 2000;35(2):162-167.
8. France DJ, Levin S, Hemphill R, et al. Emergency physicians' behaviors and workload in the presence of an electronic whiteboard. *Int J Med Inform.* 2005;74(10):827-837.
9. Levin S, Aronsky D, Hemphill R, Han J, Slagle J, France DJ. Shifting toward balance: measuring the distribution of workload among emergency physician teams. *Ann Emerg Med.* 2007;50(4):419-423.
10. To Err Is Human: Building a Safer Health System. Institute of Medicine. Washington, DC: National Academies Press; 2000.
11. Aronsky D, Jones I, Lanaghan K, Slovis CM. Supporting patient care in the emergency department with a computerized whiteboard system. *J Am Med Inform Assoc.* 2007;15(2):184-194.
12. Belser D, Aronsky D, Dilts DM, Ferreira J. Developing an emergency department information system: a case history. In: Lorenzi NM, Ash J, Einbinder J, McPhee W, Einbinder L, eds. *Transforming Health Care Through Information: Case Studies.* 2nd ed. New York: Springer; 2004.
13. Gilboy N, Tanabe P, Travers DA, Rosenau AM, Eitel DR. Emergency severity index, Version 4: Implementation Handbook. AHRQ Publication No. 05-0046-2; May 2005. Agency for Healthcare Research and Quality, Rockville, MD. Available at: http://www.ahrq.gov/research/esi/

14. Emergency medical treatment and active labor act (EMTALA). Federal Register 68,174. 2003:53222.
15. MacClean S. *ENA National Benchmark Guide: Emergency Departments*. Des Plaines, IL: Emergency Nurses Association; 2002.
16. Emergency Nurses Association. *Position statements: ENA board approves statement on joint ENA/ACEP five-level triage task force*. Des Plaines, IL: Emergency Nurses Association; 2003.
17. Physicians ACOE. *ACEP Policy Statements: Triage Scale Standardization*. Dallas, TX: American College of Emergency Physicians; 2003.
18. Eitel DR, Travers DA, Rosenau AM, Gilboy N, Wuerz RC. The emergency severity index triage algorithm version 2 is reliable and valid. *Acad Emerg Med*. 2003;10(10):1070-1080.
19. Tanabe P, Gimbel R, Yarnold PR, Kyriacou DN, Adams JG. Reliability and validity of scores on the emergency severity index version 3. *Acad Emerg Med*. 2004;11(1):59-65.
20. Van Gerven R, Delooz H, Sermeus W. Systematic triage in the emergency department using the Australian National triage scale: a pilot project. *Eur J Emerg Med*. 2001;8(1):3-7.
21. Considine J, Ung L, Thomas S. Triage nurses' decisions using the national triage scale for Australian emergency departments. *Accid Emerg Nurs*. 2000;8(4):201-209.
22. Cronin JG. The introduction of the Manchester triage scale to an emergency department in the Republic of Ireland. *Accid Emerg Nurs*. 2003;11(2):121-125.
23. J Murray M. The Canadian triage and acuity scale: a Canadian perspective on emergency department triage. *Emerg Med* (Fremantle). 2003;15(1):6-10.
24. Beveridge R, Ducharme J, Janes L, Beaulieu S, Walter S. Reliability of the Canadian emergency department triage and acuity scale: interrater agreement. *Ann Emerg Med*. 1999;34(2):155-159.
25. Beveridge R. CAEP issues. The Canadian triage and acuity scale: a new and critical element in health care reform. Canadian association of emergency physicians. *J Emerg Med*. 1998;16(3): 507-511.
26. Morris AH. Developing and implementing computerized protocols for standardization of clinical decisions. *Ann Intern Med*. 2000;132(5):373-383.
27. Rosenbloom ST, Kiepek W, Belletti J, et al. Generating complex clinical documents using structured entry and reporting. *Medinfo*. 2004;11:683-687.
28. Travers D. Triage: How long does it take? How long should it take? *J Emerg Nurs*. 1999;25(3): 238-240.
29. Dong SL, Bullard MJ, Meurer DP, et al. Emergency triage: comparing a novel computer triage program with standard triage. *Acad Emerg Med*. 2005;12(6):502-507.

14
Medication Barcode Scanning: Code "Moo": Dead COW

Laurie L. Novak and Kathy S. Moss

Introduction

In August 2006, Green Mountain Medical Center (GMMC) kicked off its barcode medication administration (BCMA) project. The decision to implement barcoding was the result of a focus on "closing the loop" in medication management. Closing the loop was a way to ensure the highest possible level of computerized support and safety in the medication process. Ultimately, the goal was to automate the ordering, pharmacy processing, administration, and documentation processes.

There was a high level of confidence in the ability to successfully implement BCMA for several reasons:

- The organization considered patient safety a priority area for quality improvement, and medication errors were top area of focus.
- A significant level of clinical automation already existed. Computerized Provider Order Entry (CPOE), nursing documentation, and clinical messaging were being used widely. This meant that the clinical staff members were relatively comfortable with the use of computing tools in practice.
- Funding had been made available for the project and was expected to continue throughout the implementation.
- Adequate project resources were identified, and teams were initiated and supported by an eager project sponsor and executive steering committee.

Risks to the success of the implementation were identified and included:

- "Significant" workflow changes.
- An aggressive 4 month timeline to finish the software build, testing, and training before the pilot unit went live with the system.

L. Einbinder et al. (eds.), *Transforming Health Care Through Information: Case Studies*, Health Informatics, DOI 10.1007/978-1-4419-0269-6_14,
© Springer Science+Business Media, LLC 2010

Project Overview

A detailed, 24-page project plan was created. In the plan, there were specific actions related to bringing the software into GMMC and customizing it for the use in practice. The project was broad in scope, including coordination with a new Pharmacy re-packaging and carousel system that integrated the orders coming in from physicians with the "fill" processes in the pharmacy – ultimately hoping to achieve the five "rights": getting the right medication in the right dose to the right patient in the right form at the right time.

The other two major elements of the project were the BCMA system and the electronic medication administration record (eMAR). The BCMA system requires a barcode to be on the patient's armband, printed by special printers in the admitting department. When a medication is due for a specific patient, the nurse obtains the medication, scans the patient's armband, scans the medication (most pills are now in blister packs), scans the patient's armband again, checks for any onscreen alerts, gives the medication to the patient, and then clicks "confirm" to finish the transaction on the computer screen. This scanning and confirmation processes automatically "chart" the administration of the medication in the eMAR. In the paper environment, the administration is charted on a paper medication administration record (MAR). This important document serves as the ultimate source of truth about if and when a particular medication was administered to the patient.

The project plan called for a rapid, 4-month phase of building and testing, followed by the rollout to 33 patient units over 12 months. The team was aware that, with BCMA, they were rolling out not only new software and workflow to the patient units, but also more than 200 new computers and 550 scanners. The logistical, financial, and technical details of the hardware rollout required extensive participation from several key players. Despite the planning and collaboration within this group, they encountered some challenging surprises including numerous herds of dead "cows."

Workstation Deployment and Support

The inpatient units and clinics used customized computer workstations for patient care applications. The Workstation Team was responsible for deploying the computers, and related software and hardware (such as scanners and printers), maintaining the equipment, and supporting users in solving equipment-related problems. The Workstation Team consisted of nine staff members and a manager, Tom Pierce.

Assessment of Needs for the BCMA Project

A team was assembled to assess the equipment needs of each clinical area scheduled to implement BCMA. The team consisted of Tom Pierce, Sandy Bell (the BCMA project manager), and several others from IT including Mike Jones, the Technical Manager and Judy Smith, Nurse Informaticist, as well as representatives from Plant Services. They did a physical walk-through of each area, assessed the existing equipment and defined specifically what would be required for the BCMA implementation. The general rule was that there would be one mobile device (computer on wheels or COW) with a scanner for each nurse. If there were already bedside computers on the unit, only a scanner would be ordered. They also did assessments for specialized printers (to print barcoded armbands) and other miscellaneous equipment needs.

Procurement

The process for acquiring the needed equipment was lengthy. The table below summarizes the lead times for various hardware components and aspects of the process.

Equipment	GMMC requisition processing	Vendor processing	Deployment
Mobile carts	2–4 weeks	4–12 weeks	1 week
Laptop computers (to sit on the carts)	2–4 weeks	3 weeks	1 week
Scanners	2–4 weeks	4–6 weeks	1 week

The GMMC requisition process contained several bottlenecks, including the requirement that the CEO sign all capital requests. If he were unavailable or busy, this requirement could introduce delay. In GMMCs, favor was the strategic relationship it enjoyed with the software vendor, Loyal Technology (LT). GMMC purchased the scanners from LT because the scanners needed to be programmed to work with LT software. If the project team informed LT that a request was on the way, LT would begin working on the order without a confirmed purchase order. This resulted in some degree of overlap between the 2–4 weeks of GMMC processing and the 4–6 weeks of scanner processing. However, LT does not have this level of partnership with all of its clients.

Assembly and Deployment

Once the equipments (carts, computers, scanners) were on site at GMMC, the Workstation Team assembled and deployed them as usable workstations. This involved "burning in" the computers with the GMMC suite of clinical software products, installing the hardware onto the mobile cart and testing. Testing had to be done on the clinical unit to ensure that the appropriate census (patient list) was displayed and that printing was set up for the right locations.

Implementation Surprises

After the building, testing, and training were complete, the pilot unit began using the new BCMA system. Initially the pilot implementation went exceptionally well with minimal issues encountered. Then progressively, despite all good intentions, planning, and hard work, the BCMA project team encountered significant issues with the mobile computer equipment. Those equipment issues combined with some new software glitches would soon bring the project implementation to a grinding halt.

Batteries

All of the clinical units had already been using the mobile computer carts or COWs to some degree. On most units they were used by doctors making rounds on patients and entering new orders. In the ICU, they were used by nurses to do charting. However, they were not utilized as a "mobile" device. The carts were parked in the hallway and plugged into an electrical outlet virtually all the time. The computer trays on the carts were lowered so that a person could use the computer while sitting in a chair. The introduction of BCMA brought a new mode of use for the COWs because of the significant change in workflow of the caregivers. The new process demanded that they be rolled into the patient room. This enabled the scanning of the patient and medication at the bedside along with interaction on the computer to complete the charting. The nurses were not accustomed to the COWs actually being moved around so much, and "traffic jams" became common at the medication dispensing machines and even in the doorways of patient rooms, as respiratory therapists also used mobile carts and often arrived at the time a medication was due.

The result of this change in workstation usage patterns had an unanticipated effect on the batteries installed on the carts. The batteries were there to power the carts while they were not plugged in, and if a busy nurse forgot to plug in a cart, the battery could drain. An indicator on the cart showed the time left on the battery, but the information on the indicator was subject to interpretation. For example, nurses were told to plug the COW in immediately if the indicator displayed 30 min left on the battery. Batteries sometimes drained, and the result was that over time the batteries were "retrained" to not completely recharge. This resulted in the indicator being even less reliable and more draining of the batteries. Frequently a "dead COW" had to be taken off the unit and the battery totally drained for two days before it could be fully recharged. This was a major issue for the nurses because there was only one COW per nurse, and a missing COW meant two nurses had to double up. The workflow of the BCMA system did not support this sharing of equipment, especially during standard medication administration times. The result was frustration and negative stories in the staff rumor mill.

Scanners

There were also problems with the scanners. Scanning is something of an art. The user would point the scanner at the barcode, pull the trigger so that the light shined on the barcode, and then pull slightly back. This usually resulted in a good scan. When the scanner did not read the barcode, troubleshooting was often complex. Sometimes the culprit was the barcode. Certain "complex" barcodes that contained both lines and squares would not scan properly. This was sometimes fixed by scanning two "reset" barcodes (on a laminated sheet on each COW) in the proper sequence. These additional programming barcodes had been given to GMMC by LT to address a known defect with the scanners. In other instances, the reset barcodes needed to be scanned and the scanner placed back into its cradle to reset. The process of troubleshooting was not consistent. Other sources of problems with scanning included the nurse scanning the wrong barcode on a medication package that had more than one, a torn or wet barcode, or a barcode that had simply not been programmed.

Another complexity of bringing new equipment onto a nursing unit is the issue of isolated patients, or patients with infectious diseases that require special precautions. To care for these patients, nurses donned special protective clothing and any equipment had to be cleaned before and after entering the room. The scanners had to come into the room in order to scan the patient's armband. Initially, the nurses were instructed to use a plastic bag over the scanner and to discard the bag. The bag had to be held taut over the scanner so that it could properly read the barcode. This caused problems for some nurses, but it appeared that they preferred this approach over wiping the scanner down with alcohol after each trip into the isolation room as recommended by Infection Control.

Volume of Equipment

The volume of new equipment being rolled out coupled with an increase in workstation usage hours overwhelmed Tom Pierce's group. Despite the awareness of the number of computers being purchased and that the scope of the Workstation Team's work was increasing, the project did not include an expansion of Tom's team. They were unable to meet the 24/7 technical support demands created by the problems the nurses were having with the new equipment. After the pilot units were live on the system and the dissatisfaction was intense, Tom and Sandy met and outlined a proposal to increase Tom's staff, described in the following table:

Current workstation support
Current support business hours
7:30–4:30 Monday–Friday
Nightshift person available 5:00 p.m. to 5:00 a.m. Monday–Thursday
No weekend coverage
Proposed support coverage based on workstation prioritization
Critical workstation
Mobile workstation *with* barcode scanner on inpatient units
24/7 Support
Resolution within 4 h
High priority workstation
Mobile workstation on inpatient units *without* barcode scanner
24/7 Support
Resolution within 8 h
Moderate priority workstation
Nonmobile workstation on inpatient units
Nonmobile workstation in training & testing rooms
Resolution within 1 business day
Low priority/noncritical workstation
No clinical workstations fall into this category

Budget Freeze

In March, Sandy began including in the minutes of her meetings that "there is no capital budget for any implementations after July." Because there was a 3 month lead time required for ordering equipment, she would need to start ordering in April. However, the organization implemented a capital budget "freeze" which stopped any purchases for the next budget cycle until the budget was refined and approved.

The Cumulative Effect

The many unexpected problems the nurses had with the equipment, combined with a budget freeze, new software upgrade issues, and some unfortunately timed "downtime" events, resulted in severe "public relations" issues for the BCMA system. The next unit to go up on the system was an intensive care unit, which has more tightly coupled medication administration and charting processes than an acute care unit has. The nurses on this unit developed a detailed issue list and shared it in a meeting with IT and pharmacy representatives. The overall feeling was that the system was not "ready for primetime" (i.e., rollout to all units) until the issues could be resolved. Sandy negotiated a truce with the nurses, promising to have the old, paper MARs print on the units as a backup source of information. She also planned to meet with Tom and negotiate an equipment support agreement, with extended hours of support and a plan for prioritizing problems. The nurses agreed to continue using the system for the coming days unless something else went wrong. In the words of the Director in charge of IT support services, the team needed "days and days of the system working perfectly" to regain the confidence of the nursing staff.

Subsequent units that were planned to go live on the system were delayed while the IT staff and the vendor worked out software issues, and new battery management and support procedures were implemented. Units that were already live on the system were taken offline. It took 3 months of application and equipment testing to get the system to a level of reliability that satisfied the project team. The delay in implementation rollout was caused by instability in the new systems and by the unanticipated technical and support issues that came with the new scanners and expanded use of existing computing equipment.

Questions

1. What steps could have been taken to identify the equipment risks earlier in the project?
2. How would you mitigate the equipment support and work flow risks going forward in light of the issues encountered with the early pilot units?
3. What are the advantages and disadvantages of the proposed support model?

Section IV
Integration

Integration 163
  Jonathan S. Einbinder

Chapter 15
Project NEED: New Efficiency in an Emergency Department 167
  Barry Little, Denise Johnson, Jennifer Tingle,
  Mary Stanfill, and Michael Roy

Chapter 16
Digital Radiology Divide at McKinly 179
  Neal Goldstein, David Ross, Ken Christensen,
  Jayashree Kalpathy-Cramer, Aseem Kumar, and Marilyn Schroeder

Integration

JONATHAN S. EINBINDER

This book is a collection of case studies intended to illustrate the centrality of people and organizational issues to realizing the benefits of health information technology (IT). This section includes two cases. The first, "Project NEED: New Efficiency in an Emergency Department," describes the construction of a new pediatric emergency department with the concomitant implementation of a new clinical information system. The authors note that the implementation was considered "successful," but that waiting times actually increased, and more patients were leaving without being treated. The second case, "Digital Divide at McKinly," describes the consideration of implementing a Picture Archiving and Communication System (PACS), as well as Computed (filmless) Radiography and Digital Dictation/Voice Recognition Systems. The authors note that well designed and executed implementations of these systems would potentially improve the efficiency and quality of patient care, but that in some cases, radiology information systems do not result in measurable gains, and may actually lead to decreased productivity.

The unexpected outcome in the Project NEED case, and the concern about a suboptimal outcome in the McKinly case, highlight the importance of explicitly considering what constitutes success when embarking on an IT project. In 1994, Lorenzi and Riley defined two perspectives for thinking about success (or failure) of an IT project.[1] The first, a *project management view* defines success as executing a project on time, within budget, and according to technical specifications. The second view takes into account the *perspective of users and customers*, defining success as meeting the needs of more than 90% of users, viewed randomly. The cases in this section demonstrate that a project may succeed from a project management perspective, and even be viewed favorably by users, and still not result in measurably improved outcomes. Thus, I would like to suggest a third view of success – a Systems Integration view – which looks at an IT project as more than the implementation of a software module. This perspective considers how a project fits into the larger care delivery environment, and acknowledges that the resulting whole may be greater that the sum of its parts, leading to improved efficiency and quality.

This Systems Integration view is not new to healthcare. The Chronic Disease Management Model developed by Wagner and colleagues, exemplifies that it is the integration of multiple domains and factors that ultimately leads to productive patient interactions and improved outcomes.[2]

In general, hand-offs and communication are critical aspects of healthcare delivery – carried out effectively, they can improve care and safety. Conversely, breakdowns in hand-offs and communication may adversely affect patient safety and quality.[3-6] Thus, for example, reengineering a process in the operating room (or implementing a new surgical information system) may not improve patient safety, if hand-offs and communication are not adequately addressed before, during and after a patient's operation.

From a clinical perspective, how may a well designed and executed IT implementation enhance integration and improve care?

- Collect all patient information in one place and make it more accessible.
- Integrate information across care settings, e.g., office and hospital.
- Promote adherence to practice guidelines, e.g., through the use of decision support or templates.
- Improve communication among healthcare providers caring for or covering a patient.
- Connect the patient and the healthcare team.
- Help achieve quality goals and measure progress towards those goals.
- Help achieve contracting and pay-for-performance goals.

What this means from an IT project perspective, especially with regard to people and organizational issues, is that attention must be paid to good design, work flow changes, and system integration. Integration issues need to be considered with regard to data and other information systems, as well as among providers (communication and work flow).

An example of the importance of the Systems Integration perspective is provided by a 2003 analysis of the results of electronic medical record (EMR) implementations in small physician practices.[7] The authors interviewed physicians from twenty small practices with electronic medical records – so-called "early adopters." They observed that in addition to implementing EMR software, several complementary changes were essential for generating benefits. These changes included direct entry of data, customization of templates, and shortcuts support for technical problems, and reorganization of work flow. These observations are consistent with the Systems Integration perspective. The authors propose a taxonomy of EMR users: viewers, basic users, strivers, arrivers, and system changers – with the categories corresponding to the extent of process change. Benefits, both quality and efficiency, were observed to correlate with the extent of process change.

The two case studies in this section describe expensive, potentially disruptive implementations with high potential for improvement. Both highlight need for good design, attention to work flow changes, and system integration issues – e.g., PACS needs to communicate with the Radiology Information System (and Hospital Information System), and careful attention needs to be paid to compatibility of terminology used to describe studies, identify patients, etc. In the case of Project NEED, it is not clear why productivity has declined, but it is likely that work flow has changed, perhaps in some ways that are not immediately apparent – such as decreased efficiency of communication and hand-offs.

When reading the cases in this section, or when planning an IT implementation, it is important to consider the Systems Integration perspective. I suggest that the following questions may be helpful:

- What is the definition of success?
- What are the expected benefits, and how will they be measured?
- How will work flow change? Has work flow redesign been part of the implementation plan?

- In current and future work flows, where are key hand-offs and transitions? These are places where extra attention will be needed to realize spectacular benefits and avoid unremarkable or negative results.
- What are key integration issues and how will they be addressed?
  - o Data
  - o Interoperability with other information systems
  - o Inter-provider communication and hand-offs.

References

1. Lorenzi NM, Riley RT. *Organizational Aspects of Health Informatics*. New York: Springer; 1994.
2. Petersen LA, Brennan TA, O'Neill AC, et al. Does housestaff discontinuity of care increase the risk for preventable adverse events? *Ann Intern Med*. 1994;121(11):866-872.
3. Wagner EH. Chronic disease management: What will it take to improve care for chronic illness? *Effective Clinical Practice*. 1998;1:2-4.
4. The Joint Commission. Improving America's Hospitals: The Joint Commission's Annual Report on Quality and Safety, 2007.
5. Kripalani S, LeFevre F, Phillips CO, et al. Deficits in communication and information transfer between hospital-based and primary care physicians: implications for patient safety and continuity of care. *JAMA*. 2007;297(8):831-41.
6. Van Servellen G, Fongwa M, Mockus DE. Continuity of care and quality of care outcomes for people experiencing chronic conditions: a literature review. *Nursing Health Sci*. 2006;8(3): 185-95.
7. Miller RH, Sim I, Newman J. Electronic Medical Records: Lessons from Small Physician Practices. California HealthCare Foundation. http://www.chcf.org/topics/view.cfm?itemID=21521.; 2003 Accessed 07.10.08.

15
Project NEED: New Efficiency in an Emergency Department

Barry Little, Denise Johnson, Jennifer Tingle, Mary Stanfill, and Michael Roy

Introduction

It was a cold and windy January day in Montreal. The pediatric emergency department's (PED) waiting room was full of sick children. Most of them had high fever and were either coughing, crying, or vomiting. The average waiting time to see a doctor was more than 8 hours. Exhausted parents were asking the triage nurse why the waiting time was so long in the brand new emergency department (ED). Couldn't the nurse understand that their small baby was sick and should have triage priority? As one parent became aggressive, the triage nurse called security. The waiting room looked more like a battlefield.

In the meantime, Dr Dash was at his work station looking around for misplaced laboratory results while teaching and reviewing cases with medical residents. As he finished a case, Dr Dash walked rapidly to take the next patient's chart...the bin was empty. No new patients were there to be seen. How can this be possible when the recently installed giant screen monitor indicates that there are more than 60 new patients in the waiting room? He asks someone to put patients in the examination rooms and returns to his computer screen. Just then, another doctor walks over to take the chart of a new patient and finds the empty bin. With a desperate look on his face, he turns to Dr Dash and calmly says, "Something's wrong, we NEED change."

The Pediatric Emergency Department

As hospitalization is replaced by outpatient ambulatory care, the role of PEDs has changed from primarily being a gateway into the acute care setting to a definitive care environment where patients are diagnosed, treated, and discharged. Consequently, with the same number of visits per year, work load has increased significantly. In addition, specialists are being recruited to rural areas, making recruitment of new pediatric emergency physicians (PEP) more and more difficult in academic teaching hospitals. With limitations in human and financial resources, PED efficiency is becoming a very important issue.

In recent years, people have recognized the potential value of information technology (IT) to help manage the logistical organization that supports the ED health care delivery system.[1] However, as discussed by Haynes, effectively linking

L. Einbinder et al. (eds.), *Transforming Health Care Through Information: Case Studies*, Health Informatics, DOI 10.1007/978-1-4419-0269-6_15, © Springer Science+Business Media, LLC 2010

physicians to the IT infrastructure and redesigning workflow using IT are major challenges.[2] Studies and experience have shown that IT has the potential to improve workflow. This is important to medical leaders in any ED setting and becomes crucial in a large teaching hospital where balancing teaching and efficiency is an everyday challenge.

Case Study Site

St. Joseph's Hospital is a bilingual, academic, tertiary care pediatric hospital located in Montreal, Quebec, Canada offering Level 1[1] Trauma Services. The annual visit rate is approximately 60,000 children.

Ten years ago, the leadership at St. Joseph's recognized that the current PED could not meet the evolving needs of patients and staff. There were long waiting times and an inadequate number of properly equipped examination rooms. Information was transcribed by a clerk several days after the patient left the PED, and vital data were often lost in the process. Administrators and clinical leaders discussed scenarios to improve workflow and efficiency. A decision was made to build a new larger PED with larger waiting rooms and a new clinical information system (CIS). After a long wait, construction started in September 2003 and the new PED opened its doors 2 years later. From early estimates of one million dollars, the investment increased to more than ten million dollars (Canadian) in the project as of September 2005.

The transition to the new PED was projected to have a major impact on workflow. The physical area was more than twice as big and the new CIS was expected to assist staff in carrying out their assigned roles and responsibilities. The organization began its redesign efforts under the direction of an Executive Committee in January 2004. Four working subgroups representing the patient's journey in the PED (triage, medical management, nursing management, and patient orientation) were created. Recommendations were made for the future state of workflow in spite of the lack of clear understanding of the scope and functionality of the new CIS.

The team moved into its brand new PED in October 2005. After training all staff members, the CIS was implemented later that month. People were happy with their new working environment and the information system implementation was considered successful. However, after several weeks, people started noticing that waiting times were longer than before and more patients were leaving the PED without being treated. The information system triage tool, Stat Dev., added additional time to the triage process. With the larger working area, doctors had to walk more, had less time to teach, and had problems in obtaining lab results. Most notably, the medical team, which was assumed to be the bottleneck in the visit process, was often waiting for patients to be moved from the waiting room to the examination rooms. The tracking system in the new PED was manual, rather than automated, and physicians had to log patient tracking into the system – a time consuming process. Computerized physician order entry (CPOE) was not a component of the CIS and laboratory results did not interface with the CIS. The situation led the leadership to ask several challenging questions including the following:

- How did the lack of understanding of CIS functionality, while designing work process, contribute to the situation?

- What are the actual bottlenecks (constraints) in the process?
- What is the perception of the people who work in the PED?
- How can the overall efficiency of the PED be improved?
- Was the new CIS at Saint Joseph's being optimized by hospital personnel to meet the primary goal of expediting patient care?
- If the CIS was not being optimized, what human and technologic factors could be identified and altered to make improvements?

To better examine the situation at St. Joseph's and attempt to answer these questions, Project NEED was formed.

Methodology

To assess the situation, Project NEED created a paper survey questionnaire. The original English version was translated into French before distribution, for practical reasons. The survey used a Leichert scale (from 1 = strongly disagree to 5 = strongly agree) to objectively quantify the perception of the PED staff on efficiency, time management, and the role the CIS plays in the process of patient care. Additionally, the survey asked for free text comments on patient flow through the PED in an attempt to identify perceived bottlenecks. Inspired by previous work on ED efficiency, the PED process was divided into four discrete steps[3]:

- Process from patient presenting to the ED to being placed in an examination room
- Process from patient being placed in the exam room to being seen by a physician
- Process for obtaining patient's laboratory and diagnostic results
- Process for admitting patient to the hospital (if required)

Finally, the survey asked PEP and other staff to identify the most important bottleneck step and their most important suggestion to improve efficiency.

Twenty surveys were distributed to the PEP team (fourteen academic staff pediatricians and six pediatric emergency fellows). Team NEED also randomly distributed 30 other surveys to nurses, clerks, and orderlies in the different working shifts (day, evening, and night). In total 50 surveys were distributed. People were asked to return the questionnaires within 2 weeks. Using emails and direct contacts, two reminders were sent out. No extra surveys were distributed.

Results and Discussion

The survey response rate was 40/50 (80%) surveys returned within the original timeframe. One survey from a PEP was returned after the deadline and was therefore excluded from the final results. The response rate for PEP was 18/20 and the response rate for other staff was 22/30. Survey results both provided additional clarity and raised new questions about the efficiency of this particular working environment.

When analyzing results, Team NEED considered positive responses as category 4 and 5 (agree and totally agree). Negative perceptions were considered for categories 1 and 2 (totally disagree and disagree). Neutral answers were not calculated. Not calculating neutral answers has the potential to diminish the impact of perceived results but will best reflect staff's real position.

Staff Perceptions Regarding Efficiency and Length of Stay (LOS)

Although 75% of team members were positive about the efficiency of the PED, 57% of the participants were not satisfied with the current length of stay (LOS) in the PED. These contradictory findings could indicate that the team feels that PED processes are efficient with the given resource limitations, but the staff really would like to see a shorter PED LOS in their quest for optimal patient care. A vast majority (92%) of respondents believed that efficiency can be improved, implying an openness and receptivity to potential process improvement recommendations and IT solutions. In support of this interpretation, 77% of participants agreed with the statement: "Technology has the ability to improve the LOS in the ED."

Staff Perceptions Regarding New Triage System and New CIS

The optimism for the potential of technology was tinged with ambivalence as this support of technology did not necessarily translate into support for the new triage system in the CIS, Stat-Dev. While 42% of respondents were ambivalent about the impact of Stat-Dev., 33% believed that it improved efficiency and 25% did not feel that Stat-Dev. increased efficiency. Recent implementation and learning curves could explain in part these results. Despite the fact that the majority of respondents were neutral on the efficiency of Stat-Dev., the majority (54%) did indeed indicate that they felt the CIS was more systematic and reduced inter-observer differences inherent in the old triage system.

Although the whole triage concept has been contested before in the literature, it is an essential first step in the PED world. Currently, the primary role of the CIS at St. Joseph's Hospital is to provide an automated triage system. Nurses have to answer a certain number of questions so that the system can assess a triage priority score. As noted by nurses, this is an important but time-consuming step. Survey respondents identified a need to "speed up triage" and requested assigning "an extra nurse" to the triage process. A learning curve in the automated triage process is to be expected and improvement could be noted over time. Linked to triage, putting patients in examination rooms was noted as an important aspect, which will be discussed later.

Staff Perceptions on Bottlenecks

A very important component of this project's objectives was the identification of perceived bottlenecks; areas in the workflow that slow down the whole PED process.

In an attempt to identify these rate-limiting steps in patient throughput, the question was posed: "In your opinion, which step is the most time limiting? (Circle one choice)." In this question the key differences in opinion between physicians and non-physician staff were highlighted. While 55% of the nonphysician staff believed that doctors were the biggest limiting step, 44% of doctors identified gathering lab results as the most time limiting area. Overall, the three main bottlenecks identified were: (1) doctors, (2) gathering laboratory results, and (3) putting patients in examination rooms. The identification of these areas is a very important step toward finding solutions to improve efficiency.

Doctors

It is not surprising that doctors were identified as a time limiting step. As in most areas of healthcare, doctors are the most limited human resource. In essence, the support staff blamed either management for understaffing or the doctors themselves for the delays in efficiency. Several survey participants commented: "Doctors during the day shift are simply not efficient." In previous observations, administration noted that physicians working in the day-time shift are less efficient than physicians working in the evenings and nights (efficiency being measured only by number of patients treated and not by quality of care delivered). Numerous factors could be evoked including the overall efficacy of the day team, the age of staff, confounding factors (meetings, telephone calls, teaching) and the number of patients in the waiting room. It may be noted that there may be an economic motivator for the evening and night teams to be more efficient as these physicians are paid by the number of patients treated whereas the day-time physicians are paid by shift. Recently, the Canadian Health Ministry has communicated its intention to move to a fixed annual salary for all doctors. Our study results indicate this could have a tremendous negative effect on efficiency in the ED.

Gathering Laboratory Results

Gathering laboratory results was identified as an important bottleneck by both physicians and support staff. Survey results revealed a perception of excessively long delays in receiving lab results. Although 51% of the team felt that lab results were not arriving in optimal time, only 29% of the support staff indicated that this was the number one problem, whereas 78% of physicians identified it as the number one factor in increasing LOS. Another issue identified with the lab was that 61% of participants felt that the process to print out lab results for physician distribution was not optimal, and 78% of physicians were not satisfied with the current method for receiving lab results. Delay in getting lab results directly impacts the physician's ability to provide a diagnosis and discharge patients to ensure turnover and to be ready to see the next patient. In the comment section, many physicians discussed how lab distribution varies with different clerks, different nurses, and different shifts. No work consensus seems to have been decided. The fact that the CIS is not linked with lab results is another irritating factor identified by survey respondents' comments. Physicians have to go through a time consuming 12-step process to access a database (Calculus) only to find out that lab results are pending. Precious time is lost every time doctors look for lab results only to find them still pending.

Putting Patients in Examination Rooms

While 54% of the respondents felt that the process of placing patients in examination rooms was not optimized, an overwhelming number of free text comments were directed toward this step. Comments varied from "nobody knows who's responsible for this task" to "patients don't like to wait too long in the examination room, so we limit their entry." The comment that was written most often was, "need to hire an extra orderly dedicated to putting patients in room." This accountability issue for putting patients into rooms was highlighted by the fact that different people are responsible for this task according to different shifts (day, evening, and night). One person wrote: "When everybody is responsible for putting patients in rooms, nobody is."

Staff Perceptions on Hospital Admissions

Sixty-four percent of the respondents believe that waiting time for admission is not optimal. Nurses and support staff seem more attuned to this issue, probably because they are the team members directly responsible for transitioning patients from the PED to the floor.

Staff Perceptions on Areas for Improvement

The final question of the survey was meant to identify specific interventions including human and information technologies that could improve the efficiency of the PED care delivery process. Nurses, clerks, and orderlies believed that human resources were the answer. They overwhelmingly suggested getting an extra staff member dedicated to putting patients in examination rooms. Along with recruiting new PEP, doctors identified a certain number of IT solutions. We have regrouped them in two categories: (a) clinical decision support (CDS) tools and (b) integrated laboratory results.

Clinical Decision Support Tools

A possible solution to the situation at St. Joseph's Hospital is to expand the CIS functionality to include other elements that may improve efficiency. There are four main areas of CDS that could be evaluated to improve ED efficiency. They include the following:

- Web based tools (concentrated databases and teaching modules)
- Personalized order sets and prescriptions
- Management Systems with Robust Patient Tracking
- Linking CIS with other systems

Each of these CDS interventions, when deployed effectively, has the potential to greatly improve ED care delivery and reduce patient LOS in the ED setting.

Web Based Tools

The first area of CDS is the Internet. The Internet provides access to multiple online reference materials that have proven, when accessed, to greatly impact clinician workflow and clinical care.[4] The online tools are far superior to their physical counterparts as the content is always up to date, access is not limited to a single individual at a given time, and unlike printed materials, the online solution cannot be lost or misplaced. Previous studies have shown that physicians have an average of two new questions for every three patients encountered.[5] Given the volume of patients treated in an average shift in the PED, pediatric emergency room physicians have between ten and fifteen new questions per shift. A growing trend in the evidence-based medicine movement is toward the development of "synthesized" evidence-based content.[6] In his study, Hersh suggested that it may well be that further emphasis should be put on the development of these sorts of concentrated information resources for the clinical setting.[7] The recently developed clinical tools section of the PED website (http://www.urgencehsj. ca) can answer part of these questions. More development in this area has the potential to improve workflow by reducing the time spent on data mining. As per Handler et al, maximum use of online reference materials can be achieved by providing easy access to the tools from the ED clinician's desktop and by ensuring appropriate access to wireless workstations placed throughout the ED setting.[4] The online reference tools need to include, at a minimum, emergency medicine reference texts, a medication reference, Medline, online calculators and other common medical formulas, and access to a repository of clinical guidelines.

To encourage autonomy in the medical residents' learning process, online teaching modules could be accessible in the PED. In a just in time learning format these modules could help answer, in part, the academic teaching needs. Subjects chosen should cover basic concepts in pediatric emergency medicine. Although complex to validate in a clinical setting, this might help free the staff doctors to do more clinical work.

As more and more clinical tools are web-based, the limited speed of the Internet at St. Joseph's is a major factor that will have to be addressed by the hospital's IT team. Lastly, links to these online services need to be placed in a location where they are context sensitive enabling the physician to access information at the exact point in the care delivery process where the additional information is needed.

Personalized Order Sets and Prescriptions

While Computerized Physician Order Entry (CPOE) has proven to reduce medical errors, its effect on efficiency is controversial. CPOE may actually increase the amount of time it takes for physicians to place orders in a busy clinical environment. Although the authors believe CPOE is an unavoidable progress step in the future years, deployment of this technology on a short term basis should be evaluated carefully in this recent IT challenged setting. On the other hand, personalized order sets and printable standardized prescriptions could show short term benefits while having a low implementation risk. This could be considered as a first step towards CPOE. Certain medical conditions warrant a protocol type order set. While this exists already at Saint Joseph's for certain conditions (e.g., sickle cell anemia and febrile neutropenia) many other areas lag behind (e.g., trauma, wound care, and seizures). Fast web-based access or incorporation in the CIS can be of great use. Initiation of these protocols as early as triage can speed up the process. Furthermore, physicians have preferences for certain prescriptions in different medical conditions. Personalized printable prescription sets could be useful and time effective in limiting repetitive handwritten prescriptions.

Management Systems with Robust Patient Tracking

In many areas, increases in ED patient volumes combined with the recent downsizing in the number of hospital beds have negatively impacted ED LOS.[8,9] To help solve the patient flow problems and ensure appropriate capacity to meet patient needs, ED managers and administrators need access to robust information about ED operations and patient flow. A CIS with manual tracking can answer some of these questions.

More robust automated patient tracking capabilities through infra-red technologies have the potential to give an even better picture on a real time basis. This technology effectively aids with issues such as patient placement and managing delays in diagnostic testing, and can help to expedite patient throughput on a real time basis without burdening the physician, nurses, and clerks with manual data entry to track the patient. The exact role of who puts the information in the system and the step-by-step movement of the paper chart has been noted as an important and delicate subject in the free text comments of survey respondents.

In addition to patient tracking, a CDS intervention that can improve the ability of the ED manager to diagnose and troubleshoot bottlenecks in ED throughput is online analytical processing (OLAP) management systems. OLAP technologies enable users to analyze large amounts of raw data through a series of predefined relationships driven by a user interface that allows the user to easily drill into data looking for meaningful information. Because of its flexibility, there are many examples of the types of analysis possible through OLAP technology including the ability to analyze mean treatment time and its various subcomponents, to analyze performance trends over time, and to analyze trends by specific staff members. As a result of this technology, an ED manager will have the ability to investigate concerns and identify high impact interventions to improve patient throughput and reduce waiting time.

Linking CIS with Other Systems

Finally, linking the CIS with other systems has the potential to decrease the paper work and speed up patient care. Linking to other clinics for follow up appointments and linking to PACS radiology systems are two examples of such integrations. The absence of linking with laboratory results is a subject that was passionately commented on by survey respondents. At St. Joseph's, nurses and clerks fill in the same laboratory requests twice: once in the recently implemented CIS (Stat Dev.) and once in the lab request database (Calculus). Integration of systems is a crucial step toward efficiency.

Integrated Laboratory Results

Both physician and nonphysician staff at St. Joseph's identified lab results as a key contributor to unnecessary delays in LOS. Lab turnaround time (TAT) is much more complex than it appears on the surface. There are multiple intervals of time from the point a lab test is ordered until the physician receives the results. TAT is defined differently, depending on one's perspective. For instance, laboratory personnel tend to consider TAT from the point a specimen is received until results are available, whereas physicians focus on the entire time that elapses until test results are in hand. In addition, managing lab test requests is complex. Test results should be handled in order of priority, but priorities may be on the basis of many factors and there are multiple steps in the process, with factors that can be controlled and some that cannot be controlled. Historically, ED physicians have not been satisfied with laboratory turnaround times.[10]

Processes that have been shown to increase lab TAT include queuing the tests on an emergency basis and communicating lab results to physicians by "pushing" the results through.[11,12] First, the issue of prioritization will be addressed. Judgments based on the patient's condition are generally made by the physician at the time a test is ordered. But the facility should have a well-defined plan for clearly communicating pre-defined priority status. Merely using terms such as "stat" or "urgent" is insufficient. Physician determined priority can be effective. Markin and Whalen (2000) reported that stat testing is not misused by clinicians to decrease TAT .[13] The real challenge is managing the workflow on the basis of various priorities, particularly when the work load is heavy. IT designed specifically to facilitate this process was used as early as 1983.[14] Key elements of these systems include the ability to check the current status of a test at any time and to access incomplete reports. One other consideration for handling tests on the basis of priority is that the test result itself may sometimes denote the priority level. Laboratory systems must have the ability to detect life threatening results and alert the appropriate staff.

The process of communicating lab results to physicians has also been shown to increase lab TAT. Lehman et al. (2004) identified the need to "push" the information to the physician once it is available.[15] This conclusion is supported by Kilpatrick and Holding (2001) who evaluated the timeliness of physicians accessing results of stat lab tests on computer terminals.[16] This retrospective audit revealed over one-third of stat test results were never seen before a printed report was provided the next day and over one-third of stat test results were accessed more than 3 hours after they were available on the computer terminal.[16] Prior to this study, the assumption was that making results available on computer terminals, rather than time-consuming and error prone telephone reporting, would improve results reporting. However, this audit showed that the perceived improvement may actually hinder communication of urgent lab results to clinical areas.

Surveyed participants pointed out several times in the survey that because the lab does not interface with the CIS at St. Joseph's, time is lost and LOS increases. Automating lab results would eradicate much of the confusion inherent in the current system such as redundancy and duplication in the ordering system, as well as identifying who gathers the results and who has the chart, by automatically alerting the physician once lab results are available.

Steindel and Howanitz (2001) also concluded that effective communication is critical.[10]

While it seems a logical use of IT to print stat report results directly in the clinical area, this is only effective if someone is aware that the results have been printed. In the event laboratory results cannot be integrated with the CIS, pre-defined procedures for communication of results should be established. Perhaps a dedicated printer should be used with staff assigned to monitor for stat results. Indeed, it was suggested in the survey comments section to provide a dedicated printer in the ED for priority labs. Communication mechanisms must push results directly to the busy ED physician, who has no doubt moved on to assess the next patient. Regardless of the communication mechanism selected, it should be tested in its applied environment to ensure efficacy. Assumptions cannot be made that one communication method is superior to another.

Recommendations

To solve the throughput problems and improve efficiency, the leadership at St. Joseph's should evaluate the qualitative information collected through the Project NEED survey. Future discussions should attempt to answer the following questions.

Questions

1. What specifically is causing delays in the triage process?
2. Can triage delays be optimized or even streamlined in certain circumstances?
3. What is the normal turn around time for laboratory results?
4. If doctors are time-limiting steps, how can organizational changes help them to concentrate on the clinical tasks?
5. What impact do nursing processes have on current patient flow? What IT solutions could speed up their workflow?
6. Could the addition of low cost support staff improve the overall efficiency of the process? If yes, where could they be best utilized?
7. Is there a better way to accelerate the movement of less critical patients through other health resources?
8. Once the key constraints to patient throughput are clearly defined, leadership of the organization can implement specific interventions to optimize resources at that particular step. Budgetary limitations and local preferences will define local priorities.

St. Joseph's has completed very important steps with the investment in a new PED and successful implementation of a CIS (Stat-Dev.). Additional post implementation analysis has the potential to identify crucial steps towards improving efficiency, and most importantly, improving overall patient care.
What should that post implementation analysis include?

References

1. Massaro TA. Introducing physician order entry at a major academic medical center: impact on organizational culture and behavior. Acad Med. 1993;68:20-30.
2. Haynes RB, Ramsden M, Mckibbon KA, Walker CJ, Ryan NC. A review of medical education and medical informatics. Acad Med. 1989;64:207-212.
3. Hoffenburg S, Hill MB, Houry D. Does sharing process differences reduce length of stay in the emergency department. Ann Emerg Med. 2001;38(5):533-540.
4. Handler JA, Feied CF, Coonan K, et al. Computerized physician order entry and online decision support. Acad Emerg Med. 2004;11(11):1135-1141.
5. Helfand M. Information seeking in primary care: how physicians choose which clinical questions to pursue and which to leave unanswered. Med Decis Making. 1995;15:113-119.
6. Hersh WR. A world of knowledge at your fingertips: the promise, reality, and future directions of online information retrieval. Acad Med. 1999;74:240-243.
7. Hersh WR, et al. Factors associated with success in searching MEDLINE and applying evidence to answer clinical questions. J Am Med Inform Assoc. 2002;9(3):283-293.
8. Derlet RW. Overcrowding in emergency departments: increased demand and decreased capacity. *Ann Emerg Med.* 2002;39(4):430-432.
9. McCaig LF, Burt CB. National Hospital Ambulatory Medical Care Survey: 2002 Emergency Department Summary, Center for Disease Control Advance Data from Vital and Health Statistics, Number 340, March 1; 2004.
10. Steindel SJ, Howanitz PJ. Physician satisfaction and emergency department laboratory test turnaround time. *Arch Pathol Lab Med.* 2001;125(7):863-871.
11. Cue F, Inglis R. Improving the operations of the emergency department. *Hospitals.* 1978;52:110-113, 119.
12. Steindel SJ, Howanitz PJ. Changes in emergency department turnaround time performance from 1990 to 1993. A comparison of two College of American Pathologists Q-probes studies. *Arch Pathol Lab Med.* 1997;121(10):1031-1041.

13. Markin RS, Whalen SA. Laboratory automation: trajectory, technology, and tactics. *Clin Chem*. 2000;46(5):764-771.
14. Neumeier D, Sator H, Rindfleisch GE, Knedel M. A data processing system adapted to the special needs of the emergency laboratory. *J Clin Pathol*. 1983;36(8):847-855.
15. Leman P, Guthrie D, Simpson R, Little F. Improving access to diagnostics: an evaluation of a satellite laboratory service in the emergency department. *Emerg Med J*. 2004;21(4):452-456.
16. Kilpatrick ES, Holding S. Use of computer terminals on wards to access emergency test results: a retrospective audit. *BMJ*. 2001;322(7294):1101-1103.

16
Digital Radiology Divide at McKinly

NEAL GOLDSTEIN, DAVID ROSS, KEN CHRISTENSEN,
JAYASHREE KALPATHY-CRAMER, ASEEM KUMAR,
and MARILYN SCHROEDER

McKinly Hospital for Children, one of the leading pediatric caregivers and research centers in the nation, is implementing a Picture Archive and Communication System (PACS) to promote patient care, enhance efficiency, and reduce costs. The medical imaging department is leading the effort to ensure seamless integration and interoperability, while minimizing the organizational, political, financial, and managerial issues. This case identifies the Organizational Behavior risks and benefits that deployment of a hospital wide information system presents. Additionally, a full case analysis and preferred implementation strategy provide a framework for any organization considering PACS or similar health information technology systems.

The medical imaging department is located on the first floor of the hospital while the department's magnetic resonance imaging (MRI) division resides on the ground floor. The department consists of highly trained pediatric radiologists, radiologic technologists, nurses, and non-clinical support.

To further promote patient care, enhance efficiency, and reduce costs, the imaging department is implementing a Picture Archive and Communication System (PACS). To supplement PACS, the department is also considering Computed Radiography (CR) and Digital Dictation/Voice Recognition (DDVR) systems.

This transition to new technologies is expected to bring a host of organizational, political, financial, and managerial issues that will directly affect almost all healthcare workers within the institution. Traveling this bumpy road to metamorphosis will be a supreme challenge; how well the department and the hospital survive the journey remains to be seen.

Background

The Department of Medical Imaging is one of the busiest departments in the hospital. It handles inpatient and outpatient orders, as well as providing 24 h coverage to the Emergency Department. Over 70,000 exams occurred last year, with growth at approximately ten percent annually. Nine full-time staff pediatric radiologists and several residents provide rotating coverage for the six imaging modalities in use by the department: (1) conventional radiography, (2) fluoroscopy, (3) computed tomography (CT), (4) magnetic resonance imaging (MRI), (5) nuclear medicine, and (6) ultrasound. Sedation services are available as necessary.

L. Einbinder et al. (eds.), *Transforming Health Care Through Information:*
Case Studies, Health Informatics, DOI 10.1007/978-1-4419-0269-6_16,
© Springer Science+Business Media, LLC 2010

To handle an increasing patient load and continue to improve the quality of care, the department will be implementing several new clinical computing systems in the near future: PACS, DDVR, and CR. A Radiology Information System (RIS) is used for procedure scheduling. The RIS communicates with the Hospital Information System (HIS) to synchronize demographic and scheduling information with the patient's electronic health record.

The department is organized in a traditional bureaucratic hierarchy, with the staff radiologists reporting to the Chief of Radiology, and the non-physician staff reporting to the Administrative Director. Communication channels exist up and down the hierarchy, as well as between physician and non-physician staff; because of the difference in professional training, power, and prestige between the groups, communications between physicians and non-physicians are viewed as being a downward rather than lateral channel.

Despite the divisions created by this structure, the department has a history of operating effectively and efficiently. Certainly, the deployment of an enterprise-wide PACS will test this structure.

A great deal of background work has gone into selecting the most appropriate PACS for a medium-sized pediatric facility. Four committees have been organized to attempt to address the many organizational, technical, financial, and managerial issues involved in this effort, namely the PACS: (1) Steering Committee, (2) Leadership Group, (3) User Group, and (4) Technical Advisory Group. Overseeing the entire initiative is the PACS Steering Committee, which has the overarching charter of selecting the most appropriate system for the hospital. The PACS Leadership Group is composed of key managers and project champions from the medical imaging department as well as other divisions within McKinly, and is charged with guiding the process. The PACS User Group has the goal of ensuring that clinical as well as non-clinical users of PACS get a system that not only meets, but exceeds their needs. Lastly, the PACS Technical Advisory Group, comprised of Information Systems representatives, is responsible for successful integration and interoperability of PACS in the enterprise.

PACS Overview

PACS is an integrated digital system that enables the acquisition, storage, retrieval, communication, processing, and display of digital medical images. When properly implemented, PACS has been shown to increase productivity and diagnostic efficiency in healthcare organization. These benefits of greater accessibility, improved communication, improved efficiencies, and lower costs, advance the ultimate goal of improved patient care.

The modern PACS model encompasses a variety of services. These services can be classified in one or more of the following categories:

- Optimization of image acquisition
- Digitization of analog film and video
- Data communication
- Data storage
- Image distribution

- Disaster recovery
- Diagnostic reading on workstations
- Optimization of workflow

PACS must be capable of receiving image data from all the imaging modalities in use at McKinly. Digital scanners can be used for digitization of prior examination film images. Although film technologies can still be used for conventional x-ray examinations (imported to PACS via the digital scanners), CR, which allows indirect digital capture of images, is the preferred method.

As a result of technological advances, the spatial and gray-scale resolution and quality of digital images are now comparable to those of traditional emulsion-based film. In addition, the ability to post-process and manipulate image data can result in improved diagnostic capabilities. The high resolution required for such digital images necessitates large disk storage capacity; a single chest X-ray may require a file as large as 2 MB, even with compression. High-speed networks are required to send and retrieve such large files. High resolution monitors connected to high performance workstations allow for the retrieval, viewing, and manipulation of images. In addition to image storage, PACS can be used to store and retrieve radiology reports via digital dictation and voice recognition (DDVR) software. DDVR allows radiologists' reports to be dictated directly into the computer using voice recognition technology.

Full appreciation of the advantages and need for PACS requires a review of some of the inherent limitations of film. Shared access to images on film is limited to a few individuals gathered around a single lightbox. Physical transport of the film across locations can be time-consuming. Films can be easily misplaced or lost. In fact, film images are sometimes lost even before the radiologist has had an opportunity to review them.

In contrast, PACS permit simultaneous, immediate access to images at any time and at multiple independent locations. Clinicians can concurrently review images at the main hospital as well as at satellite locations. Digital storage ensures that the images cannot be misplaced. Digital images can be manipulated and enhanced, resulting in improved diagnostic capability. Retake rates have been observed to be lower with digital systems, not only saving money (in the required additional film), but also increasing patient safety by reducing radiation exposure.

There are other limitations of film worth exploring. Film requires significant physical space for storage. Retrieval and re-archiving of film images requires physically locating films, which may be time-consuming and inconvenient. Films in physical archives may be stolen for the silver content of their emulsion. The storage density of digital data is extremely high in comparison. Consequently, the physical space requirements for digitally stored images are magnitudes less than for film, as are the time requirements for retrieval. There are savings associated with the reductions in use of film, film handling, and chemical costs. Thus, PACS enables very large imaging studies with acquisition of multiple images to be done in a more cost-effective manner than with film.

As mentioned, DDVR software enables radiologists to dictate observations and interpretations directly into PACS, permanently linking them with the patient's study. In theory, this can significantly reduce waiting time for written reports by eliminating the time traditionally required for transcription. In practice, however, DDVR may necessitate substantial training and extended use to achieve maximal accuracy and productivity.

Any large-scale PACS implementation presents a multitude of challenges and creates fears on the part of employees, some valid and others unfounded. It is important to identify these early, and address them as comprehensively as possible in the planning and implementation stages. Some of these issues include the extensive training required for the entire staff in the imaging department, as well as for clinicians in other departments, such as surgery, who will be using the system. Levels of computer literacy and comfort with new technologies may vary radically between staff members, and the PACS training program will need to take this into account. This learning curve can be quite steep and intimidating. A major re-engineering of workflow is an inevitable part of PACS implementation. As such, workflow analysis and optimization with PACS are major issues that needs to be dealt with proactively.

Radiologists may need to be convinced that the quality of digital images is comparable to that of traditional film. Some studies that require physically larger films (such as scoliosis studies) may actually be more difficult with CR and special efforts may be needed to address these situations. Orthopedists and other surgical specialists might question the accuracy of the anatomic measurements obtained by digital acquisition. This might mandate calibration studies performed by a medical physicist to convince such stakeholders of the usability of PACS. Early ergonomic planning may alleviate the possibility of an increased incidence of repetitive motion injuries, eye strain, fatigue and posture-related problems associated with use of digital image workstations.

Even though being filmless may be the ultimate goal of PACS at McKinly, there will always be a need for hardcopy films for legal, educational, and other unforeseen reasons. The system will need to accommodate these and other exceptions to the strict digital imaging workflow. Other concerns might include security issues such as the confidentiality, integrity, and availability of data, and compliance with legal requirements, including HIPAA (Health Insurance Portability and Accountability Act). These concerns can, and need to be, addressed by the PACS vendor.

Room design considerations are also very important for radiologists and radiologist technologists (RTs). Room lighting and monitor calibration are critical for image review. Acoustic design can be important when using DDVR.

The costs and effort required for a successful PACS implementation should not be underestimated. Early emphasis on training, contingency planning, and end user buy-in are some of the key elements to a successful implementation. Effective change management during the transition phase is critical.

Workflow Changes

Implementing a technology may be futile if its integration into the workflow is not considered. Careful analysis of workflow changes involved in moving from traditional imaging to a filmless system can lead to a successful implementation, while ignoring such changes can lead to failure or worse (e.g., patient harm).

It is instructive to consider workflow analysis for a traditional radiology system, and for PACS, to fully appreciates its benefits. At first glance, it would seem that PACS inevitably results in increased productivity and efficiency, as well as improvements in patient care. Unfortunately, this is not the case. A substantial number of institutions simply layer PACS technology over existing work processes without considering workflow changes. This results in failure to achieve any measurable gains, and in some cases decreasing productivity by RTs, radiologists, and administrative support staff.

Failing to prospectively define workflow changes during PACS transition can lead to duplication of efforts, lost time, and decreased productivity. In the current system at McKinly, radiology requisitions are entered into the RIS, but then printed out. Without attention to RIS-PACS integration, paperwork may need to be physically transported between staff members with the demographic and study information requiring re-entry multiple times into workstations or databases. This increases the chances for error, decreases productivity, and fails to take advantage of the full potential of PACS, for example, to automatically route studies to the appropriate modality workstation, or adjusting workload on a dynamic basis. Some of the considerations involved in RIS-PACS integration have been described; these include automated transfer of information between the two systems, with careful attention given to compatibility of RIS and PACS databases, especially with regard to patient identifiers, the vocabulary used to describe radiology studies, and identification of individual studies (including descriptors of study modifications or errors). Special situations that do not lend themselves to automation (e.g., studies requiring sedation – a common issue in pediatric radiology) will also need to be addressed at McKinly.

The seeming simplicity of the PACS workflow for radiologists is deceptive, and may lead to complications if not thought through in detail. For example, in a traditional radiology system, an interpreting radiologist "opens" a case by simply posting a film on a lightbox, and "closes" it by putting it back in the film jacket. In contrast, in PACS a radiologist may need to click on multiple icons to begin or conclude study interpretation, depending on the user interface. Automated interfaces that take into account the precise details of workflow with PACS can avoid repetitive maneuvers that waste time, thereby decreasing productivity and frustrating staff members who may otherwise miss the familiarity of straightforward procedures used in conventional film-base systems. Similarly, attention to software features (e.g., ability to manipulate an image), reading room design, monitor selection, and display calibration may be critical in ensuring that radiologist workflow is not hindered by unanticipated problems. Radiologists at McKinly have been involved in selection of the system, invited to demonstrations, and solicited for feedback, but inevitably, there will be problems that were not anticipated before PACS implementation.

DDVR is an extremely important aspect of PACS implementation affecting workflow. Despite this technology's intuitive appeal, it actually has the potential for increasing radiologist workload to produce high quality reports. Radiologist training, including management of expectations, and understanding that the DDVR learning curve will initially require additional work by radiologists, will be important components of implementing PACS and creating a new workflow. Emphasizing that even with difficulties in speech recognition, DDVR systems lead to decreased turn-around time will help ease this transition.

Integration of nonstandard situations into the workflow will represent another key issue. Probably the most important of these is the use of legacy films for comparison with digital images. Comparison of current studies with prior ones is critical in radiologic interpretation; and until such legacy films are rarely used, the workflow at McKinly will need to take this into account. Lightboxes integrated into the reading environment will aid in this process. Until old films are no longer necessary, the old work processes involving retrieval of these films from the archive will need to be accounted for. Other unique situations that may require advance planning include circumstances where CR or PACS technology may not be easily usable, for example in operating rooms or at physicians' homes.

Changes in RT workflow will be a final critical pathway in the PACS transition. Again, the simple assumption that PACS will dramatically improve technologist productivity (an important goal given the crisis in RT staffing) may not hold. Initial implementation of PACS may temporarily result in a decrease in productivity, depending on training and experience, although RTs show a substantial increase in productivity once they have climbed the PACS learning curve. Optimizing RT workflow depends on devising user-friendly interfaces that integrate with PACS and minimize RT fatigue and stress, which have a dramatic effect on productivity. Cross-training of RTs in PACS is essential, given the current absence of this subject from RT training curricula, and defining a new role – that of PACS technologist – is an absolutely essential part of PACS implementation and workflow change.

Motivation

At McKinly Hospital for Children, the successful institution of PACS requires an analysis of motivational issues at all levels of the hierarchical organizational structure. Organizational success depends on the recruitment of as many individuals, teams, and groups, to achieve the crucial "buy-in" needed to reach McKinly's goal of filmless radiology. Motivation, which accounts for individual's intensity, direction, and persistence of effort, must be a primary theme adopted by McKinly to ensure a successful PACS implementation. Thus far, the hospital has involved clinicians and end-users by inviting them to vendor demonstrations and soliciting for feedback. However, there are many more employees (e.g., RTs, clerical staff, and nurses) whose motivation can be critical to the success (or failure) of the PACS program. The hospital has recognized the need to show users that the adoption of these new technologies is in patients' best interests and will have positive outcomes. But, the underlying intermediate objectives and measures, as well as how these will be connected with stakeholders' motivation, have yet to be specifically defined.

Lack of attention to motivational issues has been a factor in some well-publicized failures in the application of medical informatics. At the most basic level, some of these failures represent a "hygiene" issue in Hertzberg's two-factor theory – the frustration of dealing with an electronic system that is more difficult to use than a low-tech system – that easily leads to staff revolts. Avoiding such rebellions, while ensuring that the implementation does not fall prey to every objection at every level, requires awareness of what will motivate employees to buy-in to PACS.

Training

Training is an absolute necessity for successful implementation of PACS. Early, continuous involvement by staff from a cross-section of job functions will ensure a smoother transition. Ideally, the training of RTs, radiologists, clinicians, and support staff will begin prior to implementation. Deployment of PACS requires a completely new perspective in terms of workflow and job functions. Some clerical and administrative positions may be eliminated, while new ones may be created. It is important to assess and review the existing and new job functions required for PACS implementation. In addition to specific job functions, the existing workflow needs to evaluated and optimized. The training should then address the modifications in job functions brought about by the forthcoming workflow changes.

The skill sets for all job functions should be reviewed to ascertain the job-specific training required. Training is most effective when targeted to satisfy the needs of the intended audience. It should include both knowledge-based training on the vendor's system as well as more generic training in information technology. Members of the organization may have widely differing levels of computer literacy and comfort; ideally, each staff member should be assessed for his or her training needs. Some staff may require basic training on operating a computer workstation, while many will likely be quite proficient in this task, and just need to learn skills specific to the new system. Radiologists and other physician users must be included in this training assessment.

Training can take two forms: off-site and on-site. Off-site training can be conducted by the vendor with select key users of the system being sent for intensive, hands-on training. This should include key staff members for all the different job functions (radiologists, RTs, and administrative staff). In addition to becoming "super-users," they would also get a chance to preview and critique the system prior to implementation. This may help proactively identify system shortcomings, thereby lessening the impact of modifications on the project schedule. On-site training, conducted by either the vendor or super-users, can then incorporate the majority of the enterprise users. It is expected that the super-users identified earlier will relay their knowledge to others in the groups in more informal sessions.

Computer-based training could be made available to augment the other training sessions or as a refresher. It would be beneficial if the vendor had 24/7 support that could address problems or questions, especially in the early days of the system implementation. Fortunately, at McKinly, IT support is available around the clock, although such expertise will be limited to addressing network and other non-vendor-specific technology issues.

As mentioned, radiologists need to be involved from the early stages with system selection and configuration to ensure that the end product meets their needs. In working with the vendor application support staff as well as the hospital system administrators and other IT staff, they can fine-tune the system to be most useful to them. Reading stations should be configured to suit the radiologists' preferences, as they will need to become intimately familiar with the use of these stations to view, manipulate, and enhance images.

The RTs need to understand the differences between film and digital radiology. They need to be trained to use the workstations to review, evaluate, and prepare their images. New job functions may include calibration of diagnostic workstation monitors or CR equipment, which is a critical aspect of ensuring image quality.

The job functions of the clerical staff will undergo significant changes in moving from a system where organizing and filing of films was a primary job function to one in which that task will only be rarely performed. The staff will now need to routinely use PACS, including the system's workstations and peripherals, such as media writers.

McKinly's Dilemma

Given the technical, economic, workflow, motivational, training, and political uncertainties involved in implementing PACS, along with CR and DDVR software, should McKinly hold off moving to a filmless system, even though the department and hospital's economic survival may be threatened? Or, should it move ahead, despite the potential for catastrophe if the system doesn't work?

Case Analysis and Conclusions

Successful introduction of PACS at McKinly Hospital for Children depends on defining, choosing, and implementing the most viable of the available Organizational Behavior alternatives. Managing change is the most important underlying issue in this case. Other important aspects of this case include the ultimate objective of the PACS program and the benefits to the hospital system as a whole. Some of the technical objectives include easy and fast access to images, long-term data storage, security, and availability, all with the aim of achieving improved, cost-effective patient care. Benefits from PACS include reduction in the number of lost films, the ability to instantly read films from different physical locations within the institution or off-site (i.e., teleradiology), reduced retake rates, and enhanced diagnostic capabilities. DDVR implementation is also planned, raising additional organizational and workflow changes. Successfully managing change will ultimately determine the success of PACS at McKinly.

Given the potential of PACS to improve the quality of care delivered to McKinly's patients, and the consequences of a failed implementation, it is essential that any conflicts that could arise during the selection and introduction be addressed in advance. The two most important organizational issues in this case are (1) the learning curve needed to use PACS to its full extent, and (2) successful management of workflow changes. Other organizational issues include the morale of clerical and technical staff, job security, and acceptance of the need for and motivation to use PACS.

We have identified three viable options for achieving a successful PACS deployment at McKinly:

1. From the beginning, encourage participation at all employee levels, actively soliciting their input and vision for a successful project. Teams and committees should be formed with representatives from affected departments, each charged with a particular function/goal in relation to PACS development. First and foremost, all such departments need to be identified. Liaisons from both potential vendors and the IT department should be present, as necessary, at team meetings. After initiation of the system, team participation should continue, but the teams will likely need to be reorganized and new goals and functions assigned that are aimed at easing the climb up the learning curve. These new goals could include improving and modifying the software to better adapt it to the daily workflow. Prior to going live, extensive training should be provided to all the staff according to their functions both within the medical imaging department and ancillary departments that will interact with the system. Simple, quick help guides should be developed for each group involved - the clerical staff, RTs, physicians, nurses, and any other stakeholders. This active involvement should increase the enthusiasm of the staff for the introduction of PACS, and thus its use. The clerical staff should be offered educational opportunities to become more

familiar with the underlying technology of PACS. Drawbacks of this first option include the significant investment of time, finances, and personnel to coordinate the necessary teams and tasks.

2. Radiologists, IT staff, radiology managerial staff, and other department managerial staff affected by PACS provide the primary input for the selection of the new PACS through various teams and committees. This method seems most prevalent in literature as the model for electronic health record implementation. Input from the RTs and clerical staff would be achieved via suggestions channeled through their supervisors and/or suggestion boxes. Monetary bonuses or other incentives could be given to employees who submit an idea that is used. At least one team should continue after initiation for maintenance and upgrade considerations. Additionally, as in the first proposed option, a designated team needs to be the responsible for running tests on new software and modifications prior to going live. The primary drawback of this option is the decreased weight given to input from other (non-managerial) stakeholders such as nurses and technologists who may be dramatically affected by PACS implementation.

3. Have PACS initiative be solely IT-driven. Representatives from IT will select, evaluate, and subsequently implement the best system from a technology perspective. This option will achieve buy-in and support from IT, ensure the system will work with the existing hardware and software at the hospital, and have IT provide training and support. However, the system may not fit the needs of the actual end users (i.e., clinicians, radiologists, and RTs), the system may be non-intuitive for users without strong computer skills, and most likely will not achieve buy-in and support from radiologists, potentially leading to a rejection of PACS and supporting technologies.

We recommend that McKinly proceed with PACS implementation using the strategy outlined in option #1. If the entire organization is vested in the project from the onset, it is more likely to succeed. It is important to recognize that the hospital employees have already demonstrated a desire to excel, given their superior track record of clinical and research work. Building on that core of intrinsic motivation by recognizing that these employees exhibit a Theory Y pattern – they genuinely care about their work, look for better ways to do things, and are energized and fulfilled by doing it well – the hospital can expect employees to welcome personal responsibility and acceptance of the risks. Finally, by pointing employees towards an ultimate vision of better patient care, the project champions can utilize a style of authoritative leadership, rather than a coercive approach more likely to fail.

The strongest point in favor of this option is that it encourages greater participation from all levels of employees, with focus on the final goal of enhancing quality of care through filmless radiology. Members from all departments would be involved and, most importantly, be assigned specific functions, tasks, and goals, consistent with a theme of Management by Objectives (MBO). MBO emphasizes mutually agreed-upon specific, tangible, verifiable, and measurable goals. In order to promote this program, individual employees, committees, and teams should be involved in participative decision-making and given explicit time periods for tasks with inherent, expected performance feedback. Lastly, the idea of quality circles could be adopted within the committees and teams as an ongoing process during PACS implementation.

Option #1 also has the advantage of giving employees and their teams direct access to vendors and IT through liaisons, rather than involving intermediaries, thus enhancing communication and chances for successful teamwork. A particular strength of this option is that teams would be continued even after the initiation of PACS, CR, and DDVR systems. During this brief period of reorganization with new goals and functions, teams and employees would continue to work together and be held accountable for the meeting of their goals and ultimate success of PACS. The proposed active involvement with "simple quick help guides" for all employees also fits into the Theory Y view of human beings, increasing the likelihood of PACS success. Having physician and clerical supervisors as champions instills an ideal of a "high-achiever" model for all employees involved.

The offering of educational opportunities for enhancement of the clerical staff is a particularly strong feature of this option. It is extremely important that clerical staff do not lose their motivation and desire to learn new techniques and advance their job skills. Ignoring the potential loss of jobs for clerical staff could lead to morale problems. Employing Hertzberg's two-factor theory of motivation by offering educational opportunities for clerical staff will allow them to experience feelings of achievement, recognition, responsibility, advancement, and growth, and increase their motivation to accept PACS. In summary, the clerical staff is more likely to continue and/or adopt their own intrinsic motivation with option #1 as compared to options #2 and #3 given the very real potential for elimination of clerical positions with consequent job losses and/or modified job descriptions.

Any addition or modification to a hospital's clinical information systems can become a threatening situation, due to the new technology itself (lack of familiarity), abrupt changes in workflow, and unforeseen or unanticipated changes in workflow procedures in other departments. All parties at all levels of expertise involved in the change actively engaged in the process from concept to deployment and beyond. New links amongst affected departments should be identified and representatives brought into an appropriate committee to avoid workflow conflicts. Throughout the installation, the various committees need to remain functional, but once the system is live, these committees should be reevaluated and reorganized with the long-term objectives of PACS as their main goals.

Question

Given the technical, economic, workflow, motivational, training, and political uncertainties involved in implementing a PACS, along with CR and DDVR software, should McKinly hold off on the move to a filmless system, even though the department and hospital's economic survival may be threatened? Or should it move ahead, despite the potential for catastrophe if the system doesn't work?

References

http://199.96.2.32/AHRAArticles/AHRAArticles.dll/Show?ID=278
http://www.himss.org/content/files/proceedings/2002/sessions/sesslides/sessl041.pdf
http://www.himss.org/content/files/proceedings/2003/Sessions/session93_slides.pdf
http://www.iame.com/alumni/docs/Productivity-FullPresentation.pdf
http://www.med.siemens.com/medroot/en/news/electro/issues/pdf/heft_1_00_e/02jan-sen.pdf
http://www.radiology.pitt.edu/rsna_refresher/courses/refresher_courses.html
https://www.vha.com/research/public/pacs.pdf
Cabrera A. Defining the role of a PACS technologist. *J Digit Imaging.* 2002;15(supp 1):120-3.

Gale B, Safriel Y, Lukban A, Kalowitz J, Fleischer J, Gordon D. Radiology report production times: voice recognition vs. transcription. *Radiol Manage*. 2001;23:18-22.

Gale DR, Gale ME, Schwartz RK, Muse VV, Walker RE. An automated PACS workstation interface: A timesaving enhancement. *Am J Roentgenol*. 2000;174:33-36.

Hundt W, Stark O, Scharnberg B, et al. Speech processing in radiology. *Eur Radiol*. 1999;9:1451-6.

Levine BA, Mun SK, Benson HR, Horii SC. Assessment of the integration of a HIS/RIS with a PACS. *J Digit Imaging*. 2003;16:133-140.

Reiner BI, Siegel EL, Carrin JA, Goldburgh MM. SCAR radiologic technologist survey: Analysis of the impact of digital technologies on productivity. *J Digit Imaging*. 2002;15:132-140.

Siegel E, Reiner B. Work flow redesign: The key to success when using PACS. *Am J Roentgenol*. 2002;178:563-566.

Index

A

Admit-Discharge-Transfer system, 137, 146
Adverse Drug Events (ADE), 52
Adverse Event Report, 97
Agency for Healthcare Research and Quality (AHRQ), 138
Alert fatigue syndrome, 72, 83, 84
Ambulatory care, 42, 47–55, 167
American healthcare industry, 19
American Medical Association (AMA), 57, 58
American Spine Registry (ASR), 7–9, 11–13
Application programming interfaces (APIs), 110
Art computerized medical record system (Vantage), 7
Arterial blood gases, 36

B

Bar coding at the point of care (BPOC), 73, 75–81
Barcode medication administration (BCMA) project, Barcode administration system (BCMA), Bar Coded Medication Administration (BCMA), 71, 72, 85–95, 155–158, 160
    batteries, 157
    budget freeze, 159
    procurement, 157
    project overview, 156
    readiness survey results, 87
    scanners, 158
    volume of equipment, 159
    workstation deployment and support, 156
Best of breed solutions, 76
Butterfly effect, 66

C

Carts on wheels (COWs), 35, 157, 158
Cell phones, 57

Center for Information Technology Leadership (CITL), 16, 19
Change management, 5, 25, 32, 49, 59, 63, 93, 182
    strategies, 5
Chief Operating Officer (COO), 30, 31, 75
Chief Technology Officer (CTO), 35
Children's Hospital pediatric rehabilitation, 115
    available resources, 115
    background, 115
    mission and goals, 115
    services provided, 115
Chronic Disease Management Model, 163
Clinical data repository (CDR), 20
Clinical decision support (CDS), 32–42, 53, 78, 172, 174
Clinical decision support systems (CDSS), 20, 71
Clinical Documentation System, 32, 142
    analysis of issues and recommendations, 38
    communication gaps, 38
    lack of a unified vision, 40
    managing resistance to change, 42
    top-down leadership and decision-making, 40
    workflow redesign and training issues, technical issues with Visionex, 41
Clinical information system (CIS), 41, 163, 168–176, 188
Clinical Projects Executive Steering Team (CPEST), 33, 34, 40
Clinical transformation,
    plan, 86
    vision, 86
Clinical work stations (CWS), 110. 112
Complete blood cell count (CBC), 29, 30
Complex Adaptive Systems (CAS), 66

Computed Radiography (CR), 179–182,
    184–186, 188
Computed Tomography (CT), 128, 179
Computer based training (CBT)
    modules, 35
Computer Ordering Entry (CPOE), 3 see also
    Computerized physician order entry
    (CPOE)
Computerized physician order entry (CPOE),
    31, 37, 38, 40, 42, 47, 71, 72, 76,
    78, 83, 84, 255, 168, 273
Computerized triage system in the Emergency
    Department, 135–152
    and IT environment, 136
    designing the current system, 144
    initial triage IT development, 141
    paper based triage process, 138
    Quill, 142
    system evaluation, 150
    triage basics, 137
    WizOrder, 143
Continuity Care record (CCR), 25
Controlled medical vocabulary
    (CMV), 20
Conventional radiography, 179
Co-opetition, 19, 20, 23
Cross survey results, 88
Crying wolf syndrome, 72

D

Dangerous practices, dungeon of, 73–81
    harmful event, 74
    information systems overview, 76
    organizational overview, 74
Dead COW, 155–160
Developmental stages, 104, 152
Digital dictation and voice recognition
    (DDVR) software, 179, 181
Digital Dictation/Voice Recognition
    Systems, 163
Digital radiology divide at McKinly Hospital,
    179–188
Donnelly University Pediatric
    rehabilitation, 115–125
Drug
    distribution, 87
    information, 87
    labeling, 87
    nomenclature, 87
    orders, communication of, 87
    packaging, 87
    standardization, 87
    storage, 87

E
Efficiency & length of stay (LOS), 170–175
e-Iatrogenesis, 72
Electronic Health Record (EHR), 31. 50, 58,
    78, 180, 187
Electronic medical record (EMR), 19, 20–22,
    25, 31, 34, 41, 49, 53, 63, 64, 83,
    84, 97, 108, 127, 164
Electronic medication administration record
    (eMAR), 156
Electronic patient record system (EMR), see
    Electronic medical record (EMR)
Electronic prescription writer, 47–55
e-mail, 57=60, 62–66, 74
Environmental factors, 87
Evaluation levels, 104
E-visits, 58–66

F
FIAT health system, 85–95
    analysis and recommendations, 89
    leadership, 90
    methods, 86
    project management, 92
    recommendations regarding leadership, 91
Fiefdoms, 31
Fluoroscopy, 179
FutureCare, 57–66

G
Graphical user interface (GUI), 142–145,
    147–149, 151
Green Mountain Medical Center (GMMC),
    155–158
Group Application Design (GAD), 34, 35

H
Health information technology (HIT), 71, 72,
    92, 103–106, 163, 179
    projects, 103, 104
    related problems, 97
Health Insurance Portability and
    Accountability Act (HIPAA), 19,
    21, 24, 31, 108, 111, 182
How question, see Questions

I
ID barcodes, 94
ID bracelets, 94
Informatics-based systems, implementation, 3

Information technology environment, 20
In-person meetings, 18
InptOrder, 52–54
Intake/Output (I/O) module, 29, 33, 37, 38,
    40, 42
International Classification of Diseases, 139
Internet, 19–21, 41, 57, 58, 63, 66, 108, 110,
    172, 173
IT solutions, 135, 170, 172, 176

J
Joint Commission on Accreditation of Health
    care Organizations (JCAHO), 146

K
Katie Darnell wheelchair clinic, 116
    amenities provided, 123
    background, 116
    change in location, 121
    patients of the wheelchair clinic, 120
    team communication, 123
    technology available, 122
    therapist-therapist relationship, 124
    vendor representative-therapist
        relationship, 123
    wheelchair ordering process, 117
Katrina, 16

L
Lab turn around time (TAT), 174, 175
Lawrence Memorial Medical Center (LMMC),
    7, 8
Letter of Medical Necessity (LMN), 118, 119,
    122, 124
Local Health Information Organization
    (LHIO), 25

M
Magnetic Resonance Imaging (MRI), 179
Management by Objectives (MBO), 187
MAS-NAS scale, 87
McKinly Hospital,
    background, 179
    case analysis and conclusions, 186
    digital radiology divide, 163, 179
    dilemma, 186
    motivation, 184
    PACS overview, 180
    training, 184
    workflow changes, 182

Medical intensive care unit (MICU), 83, 84
Medicare and Medicaid Services (CMS), 58
Medication Administration Record (MAR),
    85, 87, 156
Medication barcode scanning, 155–160
Messy HIT, evaluation of, 104
Mid West RHIO (MWR), 15–18, 20–26
    case analysis,
        change management, 25
        communication, 26
        culture, 25
        groups vs. teams, 26
        leadership, 25
        motivation, 26
        politics, 23
        power, 24
        project management, 25
        stakeholders satisfaction
            and retention, 24
        strategic planning, 24
        trust, 24
        virtual teams, 25
    creation, 17
    focus of the case, 22
    information technology environment, 20
    organizational background, 16
    viewpoints, 18
    workgoups, 17, 18, 26

N
99444 code, 58
National Health Information Integrated
    Network (NHIN), 20, 22, 25
Neck Disability Index (NDI), 6, 12
NEED project, 167, 163
    case study site, 168
    clinical decision support tools, 172
        integrated laboratory results, 174
        linking CIS with other systems, 174
        management systems with robust
            patient tracking, 173
        personalized order sets and
            prescriptions, 173
        web based tools, 172
    methodology, 169
    new efficiency in an Emergency
        Department, 167
    pediatric emergency department, 167
    staff perceptions, 170
        on areas for improvement, 172
        on bottlenecks, 170
        doctors, 171
        gathering laboratory results, 171

NEED project, 167, 163 (*cont.*)
    putting patients in examination
        rooms, 171
    on hospital admissions, 172
    regarding efficiency & length of stay, 170
    regarding new triage system & new
        CIS, 170
Nursing survey results, 88

O
Occupational therapists (OT), 115, 116
Oceanview Medical Center (OMC), 47, 50–55
    environment, 47
    options, 53
    political challenges, 53
    technical challenges, 52
OMC electronic medical record system
        (OMCEMR), 47, 50, 52–55
OncoOrders, 127
    background, 127
    early years, 127
    evaluation, 132
    funding, 129
    OrderAssistant, 131
    the inception phase, 129
    whiteboard, 130
Online analytical processing (OLAP)
        management systems, 174
Online health care, 57
    change management, 63
    evaluating change, 59, 60
    individual response to change, 60
    initiating change, 59, 60
    management and leadership, 65
    motivation and role ambiguity, 62
    strategic planning for FutureCare, 66
Opting in, 19
Opting out, 19
OrderAssistant, 131
Orthopedic Spine Institute (OSI), 7–9, 12
Oswestry (Lumbar) Disability Index (ODI), 7

P
Patient education, 88
Patient information, 8, 15, 18, 22, 25, 47, 87,
        122, 136, 137, 164
Patient Portal Administration Application
        (PPAA), 112
Patient safety, 17, 23, 26, 31, 33, 34, 41, 47,
        48, 50, 52–54, 71–72, 74–84,
        86–95, 98–100, 128, 155, 163, 181
Personal factor, 91, 105

Pharmacy information system, 76
Physical therapists (PT), 115, 117
Picture Archiving and Communication System
        (PACS), 52, 163, 164, 174, 179–188
Policy issue, 110
Powerball evaluation, 104
PreOncoOrders, 128
Program evaluation, 103,105
Project NEED, *see* NEED project
Project planning stage, 108
Pulse oximetry, 36

Q
Quality processes, 88
Questions,
    how, 103, 104
    what, 103
    when, 104
    why, 103, 104

R
Radiology Information System (RIS), 163,
        164, 180, 183
Randomized Controlled Trial (RCT), 103, 104
Regional health information organization
        (RHIO), 15–27
RHIO architecture, 22
Risk management, 75, 88, 97
RxWriter, 47–55
    adoption, 51
    implementation, 49
        challenges, 51
    major features and accomplishments, 50
    stakeholders and team organization, 47
    workflow integration features, 50

S
Santiago Care Centers (SCC), 73, 74, 76–78
Santiago health organization, 74, 76
SARS screening, 149
Scanners, 98–100, 156–160, 181
SCC Automated Dispensing Machine (ADM)
        system, 77
Secure messaging, 107–113
    implementation of, 107
    policy issue, 110
    security issue, 11
Security issue, 111, 182
SF-36, 7, 12
Shadow chart, 129
Smallball evaluation, 104

Speech therapists, 104
Spine Survey, 7–11
Staff competency and education, 87
StarPanel, 131, 136, 137, 142, 146–149
State HHS agency, 15, 18, 23
State's Health and Human Services (HHS), 15
Strategic planning, 24, 31, 66, 89, 92, 94, 95
Swiss cheese model, 71
System Leads User group (SLUG), 33

T
Theodore Roosevelt Cancer Center (TRCC),
        29–43
    clinical system vendor selection, 31
    evaluation and project closing document, 36
    focus of the case, 31
    IT structure, 30
    nursing documentation, teams, training,
        and implementation support, 34
    nursing documentation, use of consultants
        and goals/objectives, 34
    organizational history/background, 30
    post-implementation issues, 35

U
Useful research, evaluation of, 105
User interface issues, 109
Utilization-focused evaluation, 105

V
Valley Regional Medical Center
        (VRMC), 83
Vanderbilt Patient Portal, 107–113
Vanderbilt University Medical Center, 139
Viewpoints, 18, 23
Visionex Clinical Access, 32, 33
Visionex oncology module, 36

W
What question, *see* Questions
Wheelchair clinic, 115–125
When question, *see* Questions
Whiteboard, 53, 127, 130–132, 137, 149
Why question, *see* Questions
Wireless LAN, 77
WizOrder, 136, 137, 139, 143–145, 149–151

CPSIA information can be obtained at www.ICGtesting.com

224073LV00006B/92/P